Adornment
Awakening the
Conscious Man:
Walking the Tantric Path

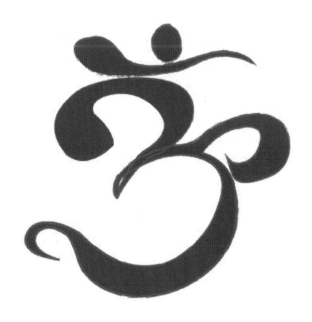

Rishi Eric Infanti

eric@MelaAcademy.com
www.MelaAcademy.com

Ordering Information:

Quantity sales. Special discounts are available on quantity purchases by corporations, associations, and others. For details, contact the "Special Sales Department" at the email address above.

Adornment - Awakening the Conscious Man: Walking the Tantric Path
Rishi Eric Infanti. —1st ed.

ISBN: 9781544046532

Contents

i

Disclaimer

Health Disclaimer, Liability, and Indemnity

Health Disclaimer:

The book, or website, or training contains information intended to assist you in improving your health and overall well-being, however, the information presented herein is offered only as-is for informational and educational purposes and is not a substitute for the professional judgment of a medical professional.

Rishi Eric Infanti makes no warranty or representation whatsoever regarding the services or products provided through or in connection with the book, website, or training. Use your own discretion when performing any Yoga practices. Work at your own level and explore your own limits.

The reader and viewer of the information presented here assumes all risks when using the information provided herein. This book, and website's operators, authors, owners, and affiliates disclaim any and all liability from the information provided herein. Any medical, financial, legal, health, psychological or other information provided on this book or website is not intended as a replacement for professional consultations with qualified practitioners. If this book or website provides health-related or medical information, no such information provided by this site is intended to treat or cure any disease or to offer any specific diagnosis to any individual as we do not give medical advice, nor do we provide medical or diagnostic services.

We strongly recommend that you get professional medical advice before you perform any techniques, poses, postures or routines presented on this book or website or before using any of our text, video, audio, or products.

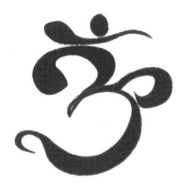

"Our biological body itself is a form of hardware that needs re-programming through Tantra like a new spiritual software which can release or unblock its potential."

~ Slavoj Žižek

"The body can become a vehicle to that which is beyond body, and sex energy can become a spiritual force."

~ *Osho*

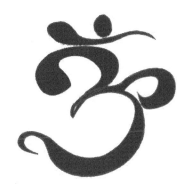

Introduction

THE PRACTICE OF TANTRA IS DEEPLY ROOTED IN *Buddhism* and *Hinduism*. Although, this practice has spread beyond just Buddhism and Hinduism, it is common among other religions in Asia also, especially in East Asia. Tantra has been created to be believed as a system shrouded in mystery, especially for people in the West.

However, there is absolutely nothing mysterious about Tantra, it is a system that can be of benefit to all. It is a system that works based on our intention and imagination. Our imagination is a powerful tool that fuels the practice of Tantra at the basic level. The imagination is a powerful tool for most world religions, especially for Buddhists or Hinduists.

The mind is cultivated as a powerful tool in both religions, and the powerful of imagination cannot be overstated in these two religions. The mind is a tool that is accessible to everyone, *and the ability to imagine and to create things out of our imagination is a gift for everyone too.* It is this gift that the practice of Tantra taps into. Tantra allows you to attain the stage where you can be of maximum use to everyone around you and the world over, the stage of Buddhahood. Attaining the stage of Buddhahood is not a chance that is granted to everyone.

My goal is not to convert you or to give you the needed solid foundation of Buddhism, my goal is to educate you about the importance of Tantra and Yoga and why it is so vital to our humanity. You do not need to have a solid foundation in the core of Buddhism and understand the tenets of this ancient religion. The good thing about Tantric practice is that you do not need to be an adherent of Buddhism before you can practice it, it is for open for everyone.

Tantra can be of great help in helping us heal from all the self-inflicted wound of dysfunctional relationships and help us to form meaningful relations with others and desist of relationship practices that only serves our lower interests while the interest of the other person is not taken into awareness. *There's a place for us to enjoy deep and spiritual connections with others if we will only learn to allow it.*

What is Tantra?

Over the years, a lot of interpretations have been ascribed to Tantra. The meaning has not changed, the act has not changed but a lot of misconceptions have been attached to its meaning. These misconceptions have given it a completely different meaning to different people. In fact, the word and what it represents means different things to both the followers and those who study from outside the circle.

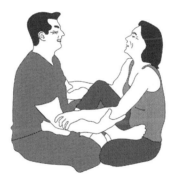

As with most things that belonged to the indigenous people, colonialism did not have a good influence on Tantra, especially as it has been considered as being a ritualistic religion with a lot of esoteric practices. For instance, *Andre Padoux*, while reviewing the definitions of Tantra put forward two definitions – both of which he also rejected – the first is stated to be *"any system of observances about the vision of man and the cosmos where correspondences between the inner world of the person and the macrocosmic reality play an essential role."*

This may sound like a boring and complex philosophical school of thought for some people, but this definition is the commonly found among Tantra follower and it is believed to capture the core belief of the Tantra. The second is commonly heard among non-practitioners or those who just observe is that *"it is some set of mechanistic rituals."* These people omit, completely, the fact that it is beyond rituals, they completely leave out the ideological side.

The truth is that Tantra has a varied wide range of definitions, and it is hard to choose one as the truest definition or as the most commonly accepted. David Gray, a scholar, explained that *"Tantra traditions are manifold, spanning several religious traditions and cultural worlds. As a result, they are also diverse, which makes it a significant challenge to come up with an adequate definition."* As Gray stated, defining Tantra becomes more challenging when it is put in the perspective of the fact that it is a lot of historical significance in a lot of major Indian religions. Also, it is known to exist in some other parts of Asia.

Defining it from the perspective of one religion or culture would be to ignore the way other religions and cultures perceive it. It is like attempting to define Christianity or Islam, when there are a thousand different ways people practice these religions all over the world. However, a common ground to know what Tantra really is to describe what it means to the practitioners, and the experience it gives them.

To the practitioners of Tantra, it is a system that embodies their way of life. As opposed to what a lot of observers think, Tantra integrates across all the aspects of life of its practitioners, including how they relate with others, how they live, how they love, how they make love, how they meditate, among other techniques. It is more of a combination of things like the texts of Tantra, its techniques, the rituals and the monastic practices, meditation, Yoga and ideology. These, to a very large extent, covers what Tantra means to the practitioners.

The practice of Tantra is built on certain core foundations, and these foundations are *highly revered*. Tantra is an advanced form of *Mahayana*. Mahayana is one of the branches of Buddhism, in fact, it is one of the two – *sometimes regarded as three* – main branches of Buddhism. It is also a term of a term used for the classification of Buddhist philosophies. It holds that enlightenment is achievable in a single lifetime. More interestingly, it teaches that even this – *enlightenment* – can be accomplished by a layman.

The aspects which are especially important in the foundation of Tantra are:

- Safe direction (*refuge*)
- The determination to be free of all the suffering and its causes (*renunciation*)
- Strict ethical self-discipline
- A Bodhichitta aim (*to attain enlightenment for the benefit of all beings*)
- The six perfections (*far reaching attitudes, paramitas*)
- Concentration
- Discriminating awareness of void (*emptiness*)

The moment someone is able to attain total stability in their study and training of all the foundations listed above, such a person is ready to enter into Tantra practice. However, it is also important for such a person to complete the process of intensive preliminary practices.

The preliminary practices are important because they help purify negative potentials in the mind of the person, and they help build up positive ones in place of the negatives. As we have established earlier, the mind and the power of imagination are important aspects in the practice of Tantra.

A lot of the philosophies which Tantra practice borders on have been highlighted and mentioned briefly. Most of the topics in Tantra practice are spiritual topics, geared towards helping practitioners attain a highest practice.

However, the practice is more commonly known in the West for the way it portrays sexuality. If the word Tantra rings a bell to an average person, especially in the West, it would be for the way it is believed to describe sex.

While it is a practice that has somethings to say about using sexual intimacy as one of the ways to achieve enlightenment, only a small portion of Tantra does and there are other vital elements in Tantra. When people limit Tantra to sex and sexual techniques, it shows ignorance, and how they have been fed misconceptions. The reason for this may not be so farfetched, it may be because when people start to know about something, they assume that they already know it all, not allowing themselves enough time to get know about the concept at all.

When it comes to practices that have been widely misunderstood, confused, and highly conflicted, the *Siamese twins* of Tantra and the Kamasutra comes to mind. These two ancient Indian traditions have been grossly misinterpreted and misrepresented by the West. When you ask most people, who have a little clue about what the word

"Tantra" is, their response most of the time shows that they do not understand what this concept really is. Their response will most times be outside of the real meaning of this word. The answer, most likely, is always centered around sex or sexuality. Many books that talks about sex has a chapter dedicated to Tantra. To them, Tantra is a spiritual approach to sex or a sexy approach to spirituality, but either way, it is about sex. In the midst of all the misconceptions that surround its beautiful philosophy, what exactly is Tantra?

As a result of the culture of learning and doing that pervades our society, we've been taught to believe that we can learn and do all things but this is not the case for Tantra. Tantra isn't something that can be taught or learned per se. *This esoteric subject can be likened to the process which led to the ripening of a fruit. The farmer may have planted the seed, watered and even weeded it, but the part of fruit ripening isn't the farmer's doing, something greater than his effort is responsible for it.*

Tantra has an origin in Sanskrit and according to *Shrii Shrii Ánandamúrti*, an indigenous Tantric guru and Sanskrit scholar, the word "Tantra" has two root words *"tan"* which means to liberate and *"tra"* meaning from bondage, from limitations. Bringing these root words together, Tantra can then be described as *a path of liberation from bondage.* This path can involve a practice, science, or system.

Liberation from the limitations of life, *weave the web of life,* another meaning of the word "Tantra", and you successfully weave this web when you're involved in and fully participating in all aspects of life. And when we say all aspect of life we are talking of health, philosophy, belief, etc.

The way Tantra is viewed and practiced in the West is quite different from the original ways it was meant to be practiced. Tantra is multifaceted and offers not only information but guidance on all aspect of life and living. In the tradition of Tantra, awakening is sought through embodiment and union is pursued through intimacy and relationship.

> Tantra is a set of rich, dense understanding aimed at enlightenment but the path to achieving this enlightenment is littered with techniques and tools which are to help you on this discovery. As a result of the inclusivity of the practice of Tantra, these tools and techniques, although encompass sexual practice, are vastly and widely non-sexual. Some might involve the use of mantras, visualizations, physical postures, etc. This enlightenment is not some mystical state but is simply the complete and utter removal of lies from the mind, the capacity to accept, perceive, and exist in reality.

Tantra is a path that leads you to the place where you can be aware of, control, and take charge of your mind. Your mind would have been completely rid of fear or hatred because you have leant to manage the subtle energy system of your life.

Many schools of Tantra exist today, as we've seen in the West and some other parts of the world, which do not have spirituality or enlightenment as a goal but see it as a tool to help heal from bad life experiences and reach a level of deeper fulfillment. The focus here is sexual freedom, connection to the body, and the amplification of pleasure. As crucial as this is in our evolution as specie, it is still not the full picture.

The truth is that sexual power and pleasure, the freeing of oneself from shame and repression, and the ability to reconnect to one's body are great steps towards wholeness, but the full picture is way bigger than these. Tantra is more. *It's about living life in way where you allow it to live you.* You do not obstruct anything. You go on the path of life and inhale when it inhales. Pleasure and sex is, no doubt, parts of life, but to reduce the merging of oneself with life to only better sex or orgasms is to miss the mark.

Tantric Yoga

Tantra Yoga as can easily be assumed is a form of Yoga that employs the practices of Tantra. It is a fusion of Tantra and Yoga. Even though Yoga is a very popular practice, and it has even grown more in popularity recently, however, it would be wrong to assume that everyone knows or understands what Yoga is. Yoga, just like the very concept of Tantra, just like every practice related to religion and the mind, is very complex and quite difficult to pin down. It is, however, very important for us to fully understand the concept of Yoga first before we delve into Tantra Yoga.

Just like the concept of Tantra and the general religion of Buddha and Hindu, Yoga has its origin in ancient India in South East Asia. Just like Tantra, Yoga originates from Hinduism; it is one of the six orthodox schools of Hindu philosophy. It is believed to have started a long time ago, specifically around the 5th or 6th century BCE, however, it only became popular in the West around the 20th century.

Yoga can be seen as a group of physical, mental and spiritual practices or disciplines. The word Yoga has it etymology in from the Sanskrit word *"yuj"* which means *"to attach, join, harness, yoke"*. However, the Sanskrit word Yoga itself translates to "yoke". Yoga is a spiritual practice that seeks to unite, it seeks to unite the mind, body and spirit with the Divine. With this unification comes liberation.

While there are different aspects of Yoga, it most usually associated with the physical aspects of it, especially the practice of Yoga asanas. A lot of people practice asanas as a way of building flexibility and strength. Asana is the posture which people who practice Yoga sit. These postures are believed to help meditation; they are postures that are firm but at the same time relaxed. Most times, when you hear people talk about practicing Yoga, in most cases, they are talking about the practice of asana, which a lot of people engage in for its health benefits.

However, asana is only one of the *Eight Limbs of Yoga*, as proposed by Patanjali, one of the main early scholars of Yoga.

1.   *Yama*
This is one of the eight limbs, and it is made up of five ethical rules in Hinduism and these rules can be seen as 'moral imperatives'. The five yamas are:

- *Ahimsa*: Nonviolence, non –harming other living beings
- *Satya*: truthfulness, non –falsehood
- *Asteya*: non –stealing
- *Brahmacarya*: chastity, martial fidelity or sexual restraint
- *Aparigraha*: non –avarice, non –possessiveness

2.   *Niyama*

This has five components too, and they are called the five inner observances. Broadly explained, it includes dos of Yoga (the virtuous habits and behaviors. The five components are:

- *Sauca*: purity, clearness of mind, speech and body
- *Santosa*: contentment, acceptance of others and the ability to accept the circumstance that one is in, as it is, in order to be able to overcome it.
- *Tapas*: persistence. Perseverance and austerity
- *Svadhyaya*: this related to the examination of one's actions, thoughts and speeches, starting from the study of Vedas, to the study of self. It also includes, self–reflection, introspection of self's thoughts, speeches and actions.
- *Isvarapranidhana*: this can be described as the contemplation of God or the Supreme Being (the Ishvara), a reality that remains un-changing.

All these are very important in the personal growth of anyone who practices Yoga.

3.   *Asana*

The concept of has been succinctly captured above. Even though it is the most popular of the eight limbs, it is only one of the limbs.

4.   *Pranayama*

As explained, the third limb of Yoga is the posture. This limb is then followed with Pranayama, which is the practice of regulating breath, consciously regulating breath.

5. Prathyahara

This is the practice of blocking out the outside world, so simply put. This is not just closing one's eyes to the outside world, but in being able to consciously close the mind against the world and all distractions. It helps in getting control of one's mind, empowering you to stop the influence of the sensory world on your mind. This limb is like a step between the first four limbs which aims at achieving the perfect physical/external state to the last three which aims at achieving a perfect inner state. The limbs are a form of gradual movement from the external to the internal.

6. Dharana

This limb is focused on achieving concentration and focus in one's mind, it is the point where the mind is able to stay fixed in a particular state of mind.

7. Dhyana

Dhyana helps to achieve an uninterrupted train of thought. It is being able to reflect on whatever the sixth limb (Dharana) is focused on. If the mind in the sixth limb is focused on an object, Dhyana observes the subject without judgement or presumption. If the mind is focused on an idea or a concept, Dhyana reflects on all the aspects, forms and consequences of such an idea. The sixth and the seventh limb (Dharana and Dhyana) are integrally related, as one leads to the other.

8. Samadhi

This is the final limb, and the stage of unity. At this limb, the person, the thought process and the mind are all joined together into one. This is usually described as the spiritual state in which one's mind is completely absorbed in whatever it is reflecting on.

The *Eight Limbs* stated above are the main stages of Yoga, to assume that the third stage is the only stage – as a lot of people do assume – is a misconception. While I will not, in this book, attempt to demystify the general practice of Yoga or explain the misconceptions, misconceptions about Tantra Yoga would, however, be clarified and set straight.

Tantra is a spiritual practice that works on the energies – *sometimes subtle* – within the body, and uses to foster and build spiritual growth and physical wellbeing. Tantra Yoga itself is relatively modern, it is a modern titivating of the yogic practices which have been in existence for long. For the practitioners of Tantra Yoga, there is an emphasis on personal experimentation and the experience, and this led to radical techniques through which the body and the mind can be cleansed. This cleansing of the mind and the body leads to the ability to break the knot *or the cord that ties* the mind and the body to the physical world.

Tantra Yoga encompasses many things, but the core of it is to use the human body as a temple to worship the oneness of life as sacred. The human body is a medium by which energies are activated, energies which will help the mind achieve oneness with the Divine. Tantra Yoga follows the *Eight Limbs of Yoga*; however, it has different asana postures developed by Tantra yogis; this makes it different from the general Yoga. *It is not only the use of distinct asana to achieve oneness between the physical and external that sets Tantra Yoga apart, the use of different breathing exercises (Pranayama) also sets it apart.* Setting *Tantra Yoga* apart from other forms of Yoga is necessary to achieve different results. The practice of Tantra enables a Tantra Yogi to be to directly experience the Divine, and to also taste the oneness of the cosmos.

> The practice of Tantra Yoga can also help in achieving intimacy, and re-establishing sexual connection. This aspect of it is very popular, especially in the West. Tantra Yoga can be used to pursue awakening through embodiment, and genuine union is sought through relationship and union.

Our Western View of this Sacred Practice

The Western view of Tantra Yoga is mostly made up of a lot of misinformation, misconceptions and misrepresentation of what Tantra Yoga really stands for. The commonest form of Yoga is that which emphasizes the role of sexual intimacy of a way attaining awakening, however, this is only what a lot of scholars and yogis refer to as the 'left hand' schools of Tantra. The left-hand schools used practices such as consuming sex, alcohol and meat as some of the powerful tools for awakening and transformation. However, this does not define the whole perception of the Western world towards Tantra Yoga. I am going to take you through some of the Western views of Tantra Yoga, and clarify the misconceptions that may be in each.

As I have tried to explain above, Tantra Yoga is a spiritual practice that is deeply rooted in Indian beliefs and philosophy, not just a way of having sex or a way exercising as some Westerners often see it. In fact, the core view of Tantra Yoga is that it is all about sex, which is not in any way true. While there are some parts that are made up of this practice, it is only a segment of a bigger practice. Limiting Tantra Yoga to this is like limiting Christianity to only the practice of *taking a communion*, or limiting Islam to just the practice of *keeping beards*. Communion and the practice of keeping beards are integral parts of these two religions, but none of the two religions is limited to only to those two things. Therefore, limiting Tantra Yoga to only an aspect is a big misconception. Unfortunately, this misconception keeps spreading every day. In fact, there is a modern form of Tantra which is called Neo-tantra. This practice is purely Western, and it imbibes into its practices only selected original practices from Tantra.

> While it is true that a lot of Westerners are now interested in the sacred practice, it would be better if they truly understand that true practice of Tantra, and not being misled.

The religious doctrine of Tantra is combines a lot philosophies and beliefs even that of *Hinduism, Buddhism* and *Jainism*. There are different aspects to this doctrine but the one that overrides the others is that we all are connected to the Universe by energy because it what made us, it is what we are living with and it is what we will use in creating another soul (*procreation*). *The ability to attain a higher level of this universal energy and connect to it is what is called Tantra.*

The Western view of the sacred practice of Tantra is strongly based on its use of sex as one of the many means through which enlightenment or awakening can be achieved. The truth is that sex is only a micro part of Tantra and *if sex is to be used, it is as vehicle or tool for the humanity to merge and become one with divinity*. There are many Tantra disciplines that are concerned with other aspects of other than sex or sexuality. The sexual part of Tantra, is known as Tantra sex. There is Tantra, Tantra sex, and Neo-tantra. Neo-tantra is the term used in the description of the westernization of the practices of Tantra, specifically regarding sexuality.

Although sacred sexuality is only a small part of the traditional Tantra, this role is a spiritual one. *The physical act of sex is only a means of attaining a higher plane of connection with the energy of the Universe.* As a result, the sexual aspect of Tantra which is popularly labelled Tantra sex is focused on the creation of a spiritual connection between people through sacred sexuality. Apart from pleasure and procreation, sex is regarded by ardent follower of traditional Tantra to be a means of liberation. It is believed that the ultimate result of a sexual experience called Samadhi allows the participating individuals to merge together and become one with the Universe.

There's a subtle difference between traditional Tantric sex and the Western view of Tantra. While the traditional Tantra considers sex to be a means of connecting to the spiritual and so used as a part of sacred rites, the Western culture focuses on Tantra as the vehicle that drives someone through the path towards heightened sexual pleasure and enjoyment while overlooking the spiritual aspects of Tantra sex.

The Westernized form of Tantra provides couples and lovers with varying methods for the attainment of sexual pleasure. This form of Tantra sex is about solidifying the foundation of intimacy and reestablishing sexual tension or polarity. The underlying goal of this Tantra is a deeper and more intimate connection between couples and lovers, far beyond what they previously had.

Even if the Westernized from of Tantra doesn't subscribe to the universal or Divine energy principle of traditional Tantra, the underlying principle of connectivity should never be overlooked because without it the true aim and benefits of sex will be missed and when this happens, it becomes a physical exercise that doesn't yield much.

The truth is that there's absolutely nothing wrong with raising sexual pleasure between two people for simple reason of enjoying closer intimacy. However, for people who desire a deeper and more intimate connection, the Western view of Tantric sex often overlooks the underlying principles upon which Tantra was founded. While breathing exercises, techniques and several other aspects of Neotantra can lead to heightened pleasure, considerable multiplication of the pleasure comes when the spiritual origins of the practice is respected and the changes in mindset that's needed is understood.

Integrating Sacred Practice into Your Life

To be able to integrate the sacred practice of Tantra into your life, you need to first and foremost fully understand the real concept of Tantra Yoga. *The reason I decided to write this book is to take you through a gradual process of how to integrate the practice of Tantra into your life.* Tantra Yoga is not limited to the stage of just physical practices; it is intended to be incorporated as way of life. Integrating the sacred practice requires a lot of thorough guidance and instructions which must be followed religiously to get the best result. In this book you will be take through every step of integrating Tantra Yoga into your life. While physical guidance is very important, I will try to cover for that in this book.

Tantra teaches us that the Universe and every other thing residing in it is fueled by one basic energy. The human body is gifted with the ability to convert this energy. When this energy is blocked or hindered instead of moving through our body and being converted to other forms they are locked in and remain in their source. When this happens, the totality of our life force is scattered and greatly diminished.

Resentments, unfinished business, fears and every other negative vibe can cause these blockages and when it does we become unmotivated, incapable and indecisive. Our lives become less than what they could be. A life without this energy to fuel it finds it difficult to take life decisions and is instead drawn in two different directions. He or she cannot fully show up for life, incapable and finds it difficult to fulfil life potentiality.

When this energy is allowed to freely move the individual can no longer undermine himself, ceaselessly repeat negative patterns, create or propagate failure. He regains his ease and naturalness and is able to truly take his place in the world. He stops thinking and feeling like a beggar who can only feel worthy when others love and praise him. This individual will know what to offer and how to actually offer it.

Tantra is one of several paths through which we can achieve or regain wholeness. My purpose of writing this book is to help you align completely yourself with your energy and so that your intention can move in a single direction. When you can successfully do this you will no longer create hindrances or obstacles to your own fulfillment, and you will be able to be the most integral version of ourselves. You can then set yourself free!

Tantra, with its sexual and non-sexual aspect, is a "moveable feast." And there's something for anyone who cares to go after it. There's no guarantee that people will get the same thing from Tantra because the intensities with which this practice is pursued will be different, therefore different results.

Tantra has an ultimate spiritual goal and also an immediate or temporary goal. Depending on what you want, you can always find something for yourself in Tantra, whether it be spiritual awakening or consciousness or the resolution of mental, emotional, or physical health issues. By simply engaging in this practice can bring about putting the body in a state of healthy psychological balance.

Tantra is focused on putting the body's sexual energy into good use. The transmutation of this energy can lead to unlimited pleasure, kundalini awakening, and heightened consciousness.

"The body can become a vehicle to that which is beyond body, and sex energy can become a spiritual force."

~ Osho

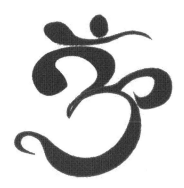

Part 1:
Healing into Union

CHAPTER 1

*"The body can become a vehicle to that which is beyond body,
and sex energy can become a spiritual force."*

~ Osho

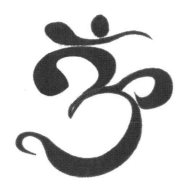

Merging Your Pranic Energy

ACCORDING TO SCIENCE, THE LIFE ENERGY THAT HOLDS
the body and keeps it alive is called '*Prana*'. This term has its roots in
Sanskrit, and it is present in almost all cultures – though with differ-

ent names. Prana is very elemental in Tantra Yoga, as it is considered to be the source of life.

Ancient Yoga texts talk a lot about this subtle energy, as it is very important to grok the energy, while subtle, controls the way we move, breathe, our senses, etc. The term Prana can be translated to mean *"vital air"*, *"life-force"* or *"vital energy"*. However, the dynamism of language is demonstrated with this word, as none of the three translations given to it, except it perfectly captures what Prana means in Sanskrit. The English language does not have the word to perfectly capture this concept.

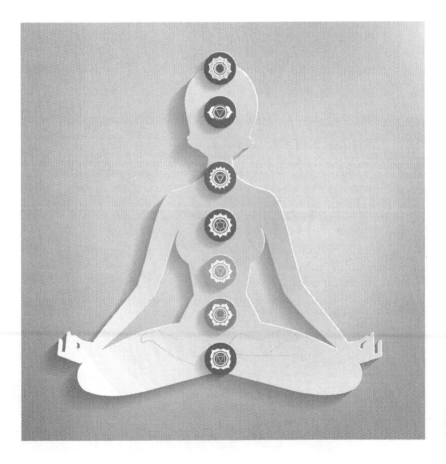

The entirety of our cosmic life and every other thing that connects to it is the product of a vital force known as *Prana*. We are completely surrounded by, and innervated by it. It is all around us and everywhere. We breathe it and live it. When we inspire oxygen, it fills our lungs and then moves to the heart, and from there the heart pumps it to other parts of the body. In addition to this oxygen, we also take in this force of nature when we breathe in; but instead of it ending on the cellular level like oxygen, it goes far beyond and touches every other area of the body from physical, mental to vital. It transcends the ordinary and causes every part of our body to vibrate with a new life.

Apart from breathing, Prana can also be received from food, water, the sun and every other part of our cosmos. This life force is so precious and important that we cannot do without it. We can live without food for weeks, without water for days, and without air for minutes but we cannot, even for a fraction of a second, live without Prana.

The 5 Pranas

In a special form of division which is done according to direction and movement, the Prana is divided into five areas and they are:

1. *Prana Vayu*: this in literal term means forward-moving air because it controls al the thig s that goes into the body from food to air and drinks, mental experiences and sensory impressions. It provides us with our driving energy in life. It also controls and regulates energy movement from the head down to the navel.

2. *Apana Vayu*: this is the air that moves air because it moves downward and outward and governs all form of elimination and removal from the body whether it be urine, feces, semen, fetus, menstrual fluid, etc. the elimination of negative emotional, mental, and sensory experiences is control by this Prana. It also controls the movement of energy from the navel to the base of the spine which happens to be the root chakra.

3. *Udana Vayu*: this the upward-moving air because it moves upward and controls the body's growth, enthusiasm, effort, will and its ability to stand erect and make speech. The movement of energy from the navel to the head is overseen by udana vayu.

4. *Samana Vayu*: this is the air that balances by moving from the periphery to the center and directs all forms of digestion of food, oxygen absorption, and the digestion of emotional, sensory, and mental experiences in the mind. The movement of energy from the whole body back to the navel is governed by samana vayu.

5. *Vyana Vayu*: this is the outward-moving air because it moves from the center to the periphery and controls all forms of circulation. It directs the circulation or movement of food, oxygen, emotions, water, thoughts, etc. all through the body. It regulates the movement of energy from the navel to every other part of the body.

The Five Vayus
Major Vital Energies Motivating Life Functions

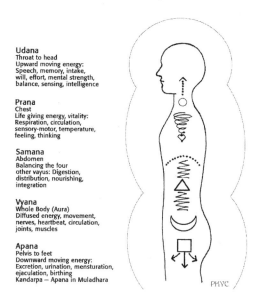

Udana
Throat to head
Upward moving energy:
Speech, memory, intake,
will, effort, mental strength,
balance, sensing, intelligence

Prana
Chest
Life giving energy, vitality:
Respiration, circulation,
sensory-motor, temperature,
feeling, thinking

Samana
Abdomen
Balancing the four
other vayus: Digestion,
distribution, nourishing,
integration

Vyana
Whole Body (Aura)
Diffused energy, movement,
nerves, heartbeat, circulation,
joints, muscles

Apana
Pelvis to feet
Downward moving energy:
Excretion, urination, mensturation,
ejaculation, birthing
Kandarpa — Apana in Muladhara

PKYC

Merging the Pranas

The body is a web of interconnectivity and is supposed to function like an efficient machine as we can see in these Pranas. While Prana Vayu controls what goes into the body, digestions is controlled by Samana, and circulation is the work of Vyana. The removal of waste is controlled by Apana while the release of positive energy is the work of Udana. This Pranas can better be explained in this form: the fuel comes in via Prana, it is converted to energy by Samana, and it is circulated to all areas of the body by Vyana. The energy produced is managed by Udana so the machine can run efficiently. The removal of the product of the energy conversion processes is carried out by Apana.

As can be seen above, the efficient working of the machine depends on its harmonious relationship. When the different roles played by these Pranic energies are merged together, the body can function effectively because the imbalance of one tends to propagate to others, causing imbalance as well. Together they are stronger and better, and divided they cannot function efficiently.

Opening to a Devotional Relationship

Tantric love is Divine. Tantra teaches intimacy beyond just the level of the common physical intimacy, it teaches and helps you merge your internal being with your partner, it creates an internal connection. A lot of people in relationships today do not really explore it to the fullest, very few people are able to make it beyond the peripheral level. In fact, one of the reasons why relationships do not last and why love fades is because the *connection between the partners does not transcend the level of physical connection.*

To be able to fully understand how this works, and for you to be able to attain an internal connection with your partner, you need to first understand and be able to practice Tantra Yoga. Not only this, you need to be able to integrate Tantra Yoga into your life. I spoke earlier about how important it is to integrate Tantra Yoga into your life, and it is even more important at this stage.

Not only is Tantra love Divine, Tantra itself is love. One of the aspects where people miss the truth about Tantra Yoga, especially Western practitioners, is that the part of Tantra that talks about sexual intimacy as a path to enlightenment, does not stop at that stage. The small part of Tantra which talks about sexual intimacy would not be complete if we omit the fact that love is an important aspect of

Tantra. The whole idea has been so misconceived in the West that we only talk about sexual intimacy, but we always forget to leave out the need for the existence of a strong bong between partners.

In this book, I will take you through how to truly practice Tantra Yoga for the purpose intimacy. A lot of people are just interested in making love for hours in different sexual positions, but it is not important to them if the person they are being intimate with is in love with them or not. Tantra personifies love, and you cannot practice Tantra Yoga with your partner if there is no love. However, Tantra does not cast you aside for lack of love, it helps you achieve it – if you are willing to.

A lot of people get into relationships for the wrong reasons, which is not good enough. A lot of people get into relationships because they are simply tired of being alone, and they want someone they can share their loneliness with. These people do not, at all, consider the fact that the person they are getting into the relationship with may hinder their path to enlightenment. That is why relationships within Tantra as a sacred path should not be walked unless you are ready physically, spiritually and mentally. Most especially, it should not be thought of unless you are certain of the person you are walking with.

Your partner is very important when it comes to Tantra Yoga and the intimacy of partners in Tantra. Relationships are very important in Tantra and to be able to fully unleash your energy, a willing and able partner is very important. The man and the woman has important but different roles to play in the relationship. In fact, in Tantra, the lady holds a higher position than a man, for many reasons. To be able to open a devotional relationship, your partner must be a person that practices Tantra Yoga too. This way, your energies can merge together.

Relationship in Tantra is about the growth of the two-people involved. It is an opportunity for growth. When we talk about relationships, we are not only talking about your emotional or sexual partners, we are talking about your relationship with everyone around you; your relationship with your friends, family and other people. Importantly, it talks about your relationship with yourself too. A lot of people do not know this, you are in a relationship with yourself, and it is good to work on it. However, the biggest relationship is the one with your partner, and it is an avenue for continuous growth. Being in a relationship with someone, like other things in Tantra Yoga is a spiritual journey. And this allows you to grow in your personal and collective spirituality.

The realization that your relationship with others is also a spiritual journey, this will definitely help you to be better to the people you have around you and it will also help you to do better than what you already do. This is one of the things that Tantra Yoga is truly about. *Here is a Cherokee proverb to help put things in perspective:*

> A woman's lowest calling us to seduce and separate man from his soul, and leave him aimlessly wandering. *A woman's highest calling is to lead a man to his soul and unite him with Source.*

A man's lowest calling is to ambush and force way into life of woman. *A man's highest calling is to protect woman, so she is free to walk the earth unharmed.*

Devotion to your partner helps your inner spirit grow, and it gives you peace. But first, you need to be able to accept yourself, because until we do, it would be difficult for another to accept us. Usually, a lot of things and experiences come together to make us what we are, but a lot of people live in denial of what they are. The truth is that these experiences that make us what we are may not be pleasant experiences, but for us to be able to move on, we must be able to accept those things are part of us. For a lot of people, it is hard to accept, and when we enter a relationship, we put the burden of accepting them on their partner.

No one can really accept you unless you accept yourself. In the previous paragraph, I was talking about how you are in a relationship with yourself, and how it is important to nurture that relationship with patience paired with diligence. When people refuse to accept themselves, it affects their relationship and their relationship falters.

While you work on yourself as an individual, you will also need to work together with your partner on your relationship. One of the most required value in building devotion in a relationship is patience and diligence. For everyone else, the concept of love and a relationship is that when it stops working, you walk away.

For a practitioner of Tantra Yoga, however, you do not just walk away, you need to build it brick by brick until it is able to stand. *For anyone who practices Tantra Yoga, your love is being renewed everyday through the activities you perform together as partners.* These activities will help you create daily and consistent connection with your partner. With these activities, every minute you spend with your partner is cherished and enjoyed to the fullest. For anyone who practices Tantra Yoga, especially for partners, constant practice is important to always keep you on track.

I have explained earlier that Tantra itself is love, and to practice Tantra Yoga is to practice love, therefore, it is important for partners to practice being in love. It is good to be in love, but love alone is sufficient for the sustenance of a relationship. The misconception people who do not practice Tantra Yoga – or any Yoga at all – have is that with love alone, they can weather any storm together. However, for love to survive, it needs to be practiced. There needs to be a conscious effort to practice being in love between you and your partner.

Caring about each other's happiness is equally very important in other to achieve this. It should be known, however, that neither practicing being in love nor caring about each other's happiness can be achieved by just trying, these things are achieved with the help of deep spiritual connection between the partners. Beyond practicing love, there are other Tantra techniques and tools that can help you in your relationship.

We are beings of connection, whether it be physical or spiritual, which is why it's an innate desire in us to crave for and long for intimacy and connections in our relationships. Even in the midst of the 21st century culture of "me, myself and I"; *we still desire devotional, affectionate, loving, passionate, and fun-filled relationships because we do better in harmony than in disharmony.* Tantra is a perfect gateway that can open us to the path towards enjoyment of relationships rich in devotion.

Tantra is an opportunity to bring awareness and consciousness to all that we do. It's an opportunity to evolve. Every moment is an opportunity for us to awaken and spirituality cannot only be experienced on the top of a cave. Everything that life offers has the propensity to bring us to a state of total awareness, if we will allow ourselves to.

When we see relationships through this prism, we can lean in when challenges come up because we are better suited to become better lovers, friends, parents, children, and humans. The benefits of the adoption of Tantric philosophies will tell greatly on your relationships, even the ones with yourself. Tantra teaches us that relationships are an avenue to grow and each day offers us this opportunity to practice this growth.

When correctly viewed, Tantra Yoga provides us with rich experiences and the opportunity to deepen our awareness of ourselves and if we can approach our relationships from this angle, we will get to the place of devotion and reverence. When this happens, we are more likely to open our hearts and resolve conflicts when they arise, and are less likely to take others for granted. We realize and appreciate the sacredness of relationships. We come from a place of compassion and love, not only for ourselves but also for others.

The following Tantric tools helps to open us to devotional relationships:

- **The Transfiguration Tool** - this foundational Tantra tool helps us to see the divinity in ourselves and in others. When we begin to see, and appreciate things in the world generally through the prism of love, we can better treat others with kindness and reverence.

- **The Tool of Consecration** - this powerful tool teaches us to take a moment before we make a decision or an action by being present. This tool tells us to pause, rethink, live in the moment, return to now, and call in our higher selves. This can be done before a meeting, meal, reading, practice, etc. this helps us to center ourselves before engaging in a tough decision, conversation or action by being ready to offer the other person the benefit of the doubt, by being able to open our hearts and hear the other person in love.

- **The Tool of Transmutation** - in relationships, this tool teaches us to look for the positive in a challenging situation, to turn the situation around for the better. Transmutation teaches us to ask our friends, relatives, lovers, or partners, what is the positive thing that we can take away from this argument that we just had? What can we learn so we do not find ourselves in this same pit next time? If we face the same situation next time, what can we do differently?

By committing to explore a difficult situation in this manner, we do away with finger pointing and instead focus on the opportunity to become better and grow closer. Transmutation not only teaches us that an important and beautiful lesson exist in every situation but it also teaches us to focus on it.

Healing Sexual Wounds

More than we care to admit or more than the statistics are ever going to say, a lot of people in relationships suffer from sexual wounds. Similarly, a lot of people who are not in any relationship have suffered sexual wounds or trauma and most times, it led to the end of their previous relationship. A lot of people have suffered and still from sexual wounds. Women more than men, have been proven to be the biggest victims of sexual wounds.

This is not to mean that men do not suffer from sexual wounds too, but women fall victim more. Statistics put it that one in four women experience sexual trauma, and one in five women report being raped, this is not to talk about a lot of people who do not speak out for the fear of being shamed. Unfortunately, there is not enough being done to help victims. Suffering from a sexual wound can greatly affect future sexual experiences of an individual. In fact, a lot of people who have suffered from sexual wounds find it hard to move beyond it, and a lot of them just avoid sexual encounters altogether.

In the case where they cannot avoid it, they do not get the best experience from their partners. To get a good sexual experience from your partner, you need to understand your body and be able to guide your partner into this understanding your body too. No one deserves to experience sexual wounds, and no one deserves to suffer from the aftermath of it.

Tantra Yoga offers the best form of healing for people who have suffered from sexual wounds. There are many ways therapists propose that people can get over sexual traumas and wounds, however, these methods do not guarantee permanent healing. For instance, someone that was abused as a kid may find it hard to forget the childhood experiences and move forward. Usually, no matter how hard they try, the memory still comes back to haunt them. With the help of Tantra Yoga, an individual can move away from the nasty sexual experiences they had in the past and move on with their lives. Of course, healing takes time and it takes effort, but it will be worth it eventually.

I have explained the importance of accepting yourself earlier, and it is also very important when someone is trying to heal too. Our present self is the culmination of our past experiences, and there is no need to deny this. Denying it or feeling pity and ashamed will hinder the healing process. When you meet a woman, who is not comfortable among men or a man is not comfortable among women, it is probably because of some things they have experienced in the past. The first process is knowing that the experience you had does not define you, and therefore, you need to accept it as part of your past.

The reason why people try to deny their experiences is because they do not want to feel the pain, which is just normal. However, feeling the pain is part of the healing process. Let's take for instance that while running from a beast you get injured, it is only normal for you to ignore the pain and keep running for you to survive. This is what surviving a sexual wound is for a lot of people, they ignore it and run from it. However, if you do not take the time to pause and treat your wound, you may never heal. Your human instinct may tell you to keep running, because the moment you stop running, you start to feel the pain, but you cannot treat yourself unless you stop running.

There are many ways sexual wounds affect the people in their relationship and most especially in their act of love making. The most important and general way it affects people is that it takes the fun out of it, and it may lead to them having sex just to please their partner. Sexual intimacy is beyond just the physical penetration, it is an act of releasing energies by both partners; it is a spiritual act in Tantra. For someone who can get past his or her wounds, it would be hard to achieve enlightenment through sexual intimacy. Not only this, it would also be very hard for the person to fully explore the limitless options that Tantra Yoga allows you with sexual intimacy.

After the first process of accepting what had happened, and feeling the pain you had avoided for a long time. The next thing is to be open with your partner, if you are in a relationship, and let them know about what had happened and your struggles with it afterwards. And this stage emphasizes what I had said earlier about the need to be in a relationship with someone you truly connect with and not just anybody that is available.

Carrying your partner along, your partner should be able to help you with the healing process; they should be willing to help you reclaim what you had lost. Partners should work as healers for each other. *One of the purposes of being in a relationship is to be able to create light for each other, light the part through darkness for each other.* This way it would be easier for anyone to get through sexual wounds or any kind of wound. The role which your partner plays in the healing process is very important, but that does not mean that someone who is not in a relationship cannot go through the healing process too. Healing is not for select people, as long as you can accept what happened to you and immerse yourself in the healing processes of Tantra, you can be healed of your past traumas.

Instead of the negativity that feeds your mind and the regrets that you may be subjecting yourself to, you need to replace those things with positive thoughts. Our society has a way of shaming victims of sexual wounds and making it feel like it was their fault it happened in the first place. Research has however shown that this is not true, so you need not regret about what you could or could not have done to avoid it. What you need to do instead is to replace meditation and spiritual contemplation. Positivity always wins over negativity. When you allow the negative thoughts to creep into your mind, it would be like you are sabotaging your healing process yourself. It is not your fault that negative thoughts are coming, but for you to fully heal, you need to be able to shut them out. The most effective way is to know that there is nothing at all you could have done to change what happened, therefore, it is not your fault.

Popular Tantra Yogi *Psalm Isadora* recommends a meditating method called KISS:

- **K: Kinetic**
  In the words of *Psalm Isadora*, "Tantra is about tapping into and embracing our inherent sexual energy."

- **I: Intimacy**
  Intimacy is one of the core of Tantra, intimacy with your

partner, intimacy with your inner self and intimacy with the Divine. The principles of Tantra can help you create a deeper intimacy with your partner. It can also help you create a deep connection which she calls "heart connection through mindful sex".

- **S: Slow Down:**

  People tend to rush the process of love making, but slow down can really be helpful in that helps you be more present. Also, it helps you pay more attention to the feelings and the what may be the need of both of you.

- **S: Sensuality:**

  Sensuality is very important in that it helps you to be more in tune with your body and that of your partner. She said it "will allow you to feel more in your heart, body and soul".

She also recommends ways you can incorporate Tantric sex in your life as sexual partners.

1. **Avoid judgement:**

   There are many ways we judge during the art of lovemaking, sometimes, we judge our partner for their style, some other times, we judge ourselves for not doing enough. These things get amplified when we are trying something new with our intercourse. However, for us to get the best out of it, it is important to go into it without judgement, just enjoy it and flow with it.

2. **Breathe together:**

   Practice bliss breathe his is also known as Bhairavi Kriya in Hindu, it is a method in Tantra that allows the practitioner to use "breath and visualization to mentally direct the essence of sexual energy upwards toward the center above the crown of the head, wherein resides the Divine presence." This definition given by Swami Ayyappa Giri, et al. may feel too big.

   However, the basic thing about bliss breathe is that it makes you feel closer to your partner, and it enables you to have a deeper Tantra experience. To try it, Psalm Isadora advised that the partner should constrict the back of their throats and take long, slow deep breaths their nose. The partners can try to inhale and exhale together, in the same calculated pace their intercourse.

3. **Make eye contact:**

   Eye contact is a very important aspect of Tantra Yoga. For a lot of couples, the whole point of intimacy is to be naked and to engage in sexual intercourse. This, however, does not capture all about sexual intercourse, it only achieves physical intimacy and noting more. One of the ways to achieve more than just physical intimacy with your partner is to make eyes contact. When we talk about making eye contact, we are not just talking about looking at each other in the eye at every opportunity gotten, we are talking about the ability to see through each other's eyes. Looking into the eyes of your partner allows you to see into their soul and see into the recesses of their minds. Everyone knows that the eyes are the windows to the soul. Holding eye contact with your partner will let you see deeply inside deeply your partner.

4. **Try feather-light touching:**

    Feather -light touching is an effective way of caressing your
    partner, it is one of the fore play techniques in Tantra. Feath-
    er-light touching can arouse your partner and create sexual
    tension between the two of you. Feather light touching can
    be done when you gently run your finger nails through stra-
    tegic places on your partner's skin; it could be running your
    finger nails up and down his or her arms, neck, etc.

It is common knowledge that one of the most challenging tasks
that anybody would face, even for the best psychotherapists, is that of
how to heal sexual wounds. The good news is that the emergence of
Pranic healing has provided us with effective tools to deal with it.

There are two fundamental principles that guides Pranic healing,
one is the law of self-recovery and the other is the law of Prana or
life-force. The first law teaches that the human body possess an innate ability to heal itself with time. This explains what hemorrhage
from a body cut will stop after a while because of a blood clot. It also
explains while the injury heals itself after some days. Therefore,
cough and cold will disappear after a while because it is the body's
natural way of healing itself. *The law of Prana teaches that it takes a
Prana or life-force for life to exist and without it there's no life.*

What Pranic healing does is to speed up this natural healing process by channeling Prana into the affected area or part. Prana plays
the role of a catalyst in the reaction of life thus hastening it. Pranic
healing works on both the physical body and the bioplasmic body.
The bioplasmic body is also known as energy body, aura or the bio-
electromagnetic field.

While only few people can perceive the bioplasmic body, we all can feel the physical body. There's a link between the bioplasmic and the physical body. Illnesses, diseases, wounds work in a way they affect the aura or bioplasmic body first before it is manifested on the physical body. These wounds come in the form of energy disruptions which negatively affects the body.

Pranic healing helps to balance this energy and this Prana is first absorbed into the bioplasmic body before it is transferred to the physical body. This brings about a harmonious or balanced state of wellbeing. Pranic healing which is also known by other names faith healing, psychic healing, and therapeutic touch provides the body with revitalizing and renewing energy to heal itself from all forms of wound, whether it be mental, emotional or physical.

Pranic healing can help heal your diseases and sicknesses no matter how deep and painful it is. This healing is not restricted to individuals with physical injuries, people can also, by practicing Prana, be healed from all manner of sexual wounds so that they can experience physical and emotional wellness.

Deepening Your Personal Tantric Practice

Tantra practice like many of the esoteric tradition is based on the principles that the higher you go the better you become. Tantra practice has *an ultimate goal, a long-term goal* and *a short-term goal*. If you decide to concern yourself with using Tantra to achieve immediate benefits, to resolve temporary health and life issues, then that's what you will get — a life that is healthy and psychologically balanced.

Everybody actually begins Tantra from this point but while some may take it up a notch, others are contented with the immediate gains. One thing you must understand is that there are benefits that can only be accessed from a higher level of Tantra practice. So, let's talks about what you stand to gain if you deepen your Tantric practice.

A beyond the surface, Tantra practice takes you beyond the boundary of ordinary sexual ecstasy to a place where you transcend this normal state. The normal sexual state is limited by the emotional and physical blockages in the body. Tantra practice has a way of releasing these blockages and freeing you from its attendant issues. Tantra increase your body's vibrational energy and leads you to a place where you can experience a blissful state of proper awakening.

A deeper level of Tantra practice also opens you to deep intimacy and love, something that you may not be able to access on an ordinary level.

It's believed that some of the basis for weak relationships are uncontrollable desires, lack of deeper intimacy, and the urge for personal fulfillment. When these issues are resolved, the individual is well on his way to enjoying a strong and deep intimacy with a healthy bond. So, if you're serious about deepening the bond of your relationship then you should not only consider Tantra practice but also make effort to deepen it.

We've seen that energies come from food, water, air and every other means through which things get into our body. Apart from the energies lost through the process of maintaining the body, there are other ways by which these energies are being lost, dissipated, and wasted. If these wastage activities can be stopped and the holes plugged, the individual will become powerful both emotional and mentally.

A deepened level of Tantra practice which helps to conserve your energy instead of draining it opens you up to enjoying a strong mental and emotional personage.

There's a whole lot that we can enjoy from Tantra and its western version Neo-tantra. The world is full of souls who have been raised in repressive and denigrating atmosphere and who need healing for themselves and others only if they will learn to manage their life force.

The ancient practice of Tantra combines meditation, breath, sound, movement, and bodywork to open the body's energy system. This makes it possible for dormant energy to circulate round the body, loosening and unblocking all restrictions in the process. This helps to transform and heal the body of any wound, illness, sickness that it has. The individual experiences life shifts, profound emotional and physical improvements, and deeper relationships.

When you're free of these trauma, stress and constrictions, you are better positioned to grow to your fullest potential and become the best version of yourself that you can be.

With Tantra, you can learn new ways of communicating and relating with yourself and others. You can learn to relate better with yourself and others and treat people with care, respect and good intention.

It doesn't matter how deep or how long your sexual abuse has tormented you, you can be free completely from its wounds when you embrace the healing power of Pranic Yoga. You can live a more loving, passionate, caring, and fulfilled life.

Tantra Exercises

The usefulness of Tantra cuts across the physical, mental and even the spiritual realms. A lot of the information that flies around the in the Western world is that Tantra is basically about having long and exhaustive sexual intercourse with a partner, in different positions. This is nothing but misinformation. *Tantra is a sacred practice that helps us achieve inner piece, an outward glow and leads us to the stage of spiritual enlightenment.*

Tantra helps us connect with our body, our soul and our inner spirit. Now, my statement should not be misunderstood. Saying that Tantra is sacred does not mean that sex is filthy and Tantra does not identify with it, no. In Tantra, the act that is commonly known as 'sex' to a lot of people is more appropriately called the act of 'making love'. Love making itself is a sacred practice that does not only lead to physical pleasure, it also leads to spiritual enlightenment. Therefore, love making is a part in the big body of Tantra.

Because of the way the world is structured, a lot of people suffer from the hands of those whom they trust. The world is structured in a partial way where those who seem to have the littlest of power can lord it over those they feel are powerless. That is why reports of sexual abuse are rife, especially the sexual abuse of kids who are too small to fight back. A lot of these cases do not only come from strangers, many of victims of sexual abuse were abused by people they knew very well; their parents, siblings, teachers, etc. Being abused in this way takes a psychological toll on the victims, and they do not often know how to move beyond the incident(s). It even becomes tougher when the abuser is someone known very well to the victim, they sense to lose all sense of trust in people.

A lot of other people suffer from loss, the loss of a loved one or something dear, and they often find it hard to heal. The healing process required after a major trauma, or any trauma whatsoever, is one of the most difficult things to do. The difficulty in healing is often overlooked by a lot of people, a lot of people do not allow themselves to go through the process of healing at all.

To be able to heal, you first must be vulnerable; to surrender yourself and experience the pain. It is in being able to feel the pain that you can free yourself what you have been holding on to. People who have experienced traumatic incidents often like to forget it and pretend like it never happened. While this may seem like an easy way out, however, the truth is that you are still in denial, and you are just a step away from breaking down at any time.

Of course, the process of healing goes beyond just freeing yourself and allowing yourself to feel the pain, it takes time and strength to go through the whole process. The practice of Tantra has, over the years, helped people deal with trauma, and it has been able to delicately guide them through the healing process and reclaiming their body. Healing, of course, involves being able to reclaim your body, and accepting your past as part of the things you have experienced.

The practice of Tantra is in itself, about the expansion of energy within the body of a practitioner, the world itself means "energy expansion". The practices of Tantra you get connected with your body, this can be achieved through the use of your breath to integrate other parts of your body like the heart, mind, body and sexuality. Just like I have said earlier, it helps you reclaim your body, eliminating the toxic things that you may have stored up over time. Similarly, it helps you awaken the energies that may have been sleeping in your body; it helps you awaken your body systemically.

Usually, when people experience a trauma, it affects their connection with people and the way they interact with others around them. With the help of Tantra, it becomes easier to move past this and have a better connection with people.

The first step healing is to release yourself, without this very little success – *if any at all – can be achieved.* Tantra itself does not have a magic wand that makes the trauma disappear with the use of a magic mantra. The process of healing, and awakening your body in Tantra involves a deliberate effort from the individual. Healing requires courage and bravery, because even the best of us would prefer to hide from our demons instead of facing them. Of course, coming out to face your demons is not an easy thing to do, a lot of people would see it as a suicide mission, or being unnecessarily stupid. The real word to use to describe facing your demons is, however, courage. Your courage is commendable!

More than we often care to admit, sexual trauma is very prevalent in our society. A lot of people in the Western world like to be assume that sexual assault is only prevalent in developing countries. However, research has shown that nearly 1 in every 5 women reported to have been raped once or more; that is about 18% of women. Also, 13% of women reported sexual coercion at some point in their lives. This research was carried out by CDC in 2012.

In another study, about 43% of women experience sexual dysfunction. These researches and others clearly make it obvious that a lot of women are going through sexual trauma. To add to the experiences of these women are men who were also abused as kids. Other causes of sexual problems could emotional, such as, sexual rejection by a partner, emotional pressure, verbal abuse, low self-esteem, etc.

Most of these emotional issues are, perhaps, not spoken about enough, thereby, the victims are made to live with the trauma for a long time – if not throughout their entire lives.

Preparing for Healing

There is the need to prepare for your healing before you even start the journey. Just like I explained earlier, healing is not at all an easy process, it could be tough. Making a tough decision is usually very hard, it takes courage and a very good plan to be able to engage with it. For instance, people in abusive relationship know that the relationship is bad, very bad for their physical and mental wellbeing, nonetheless, they find it hard to leave. It can also be likened to trying to quit a habit, it is not something that can be done by just wanting to do it.

The first step in preparation is to *set an intention*. Setting an intention allows you to prepare the things around you, especially your environment, to best support your healing process. This step is very important in helping you remove toxicity and things that may hinder your healing.

Setting an intention is like having a plan or a goal spawned from your heart. If you are leaving your house in the morning, but you have no plan as to how you intend to spend your day, you would end up doing whatever comes your way and achieving very little. To have a plan about how your day would be is to set an intention. Same thing applies to the process of healing. Before you start the process, you should have an idea of what you expect from it, what the end goal is supposed to be.

> You need to set an intention to heal. After setting an intention, it is important to keep it at the forefront of your mind. This will help you always keep your mind on the reason why you start the process in the first place. A lot of times, things may get so confusing, and we may easily forget what your intention is in the first place.

It is very important to have your intentions committed to memory. It is very easy to lose control and forget the reason why you started the journey. Sometimes, things may get overwhelming and you may feel like the whole process is not really worth the stress. At such times, being able to remind yourself of your intentions would keep you going. It is often advisable for people to write it out. Writing messages out and sticking them to the wall or anywhere you can easily see them would be of great help to you.

Going through these messages, you would always find a reason to continue with your journey. It is important for you to write about your journey as you go, may be get a journal. Apart from the fact that writing would help you pour out your soul the way you cannot to anyone else, it would also give you the opportunity for you to evaluate your journey periodically and appreciate how far you have come. Sometimes, when we are healing, we may not know that we have achieved great milestones. However, writing down your development at each stage would help you trust the process more.

> The second step is to connect feelings with sensations. It is at this stage that you are able to learn how to disengage from the toxic stories and memories that have been stored up or that your brain tells you. When you can do this, then you would be able to stay in present with the feelings. It also helps you to be able to go through them with ease and openness.

Ideally, the brain is built to look out for you, to tell you when there is an impending danger. However, in some cases, the stories your brain tells you would only make things worse. Sometimes, you have to stop listening to your brains and focus on the sensation you feel in your body. For instance, when there is cold, the sensation you would feel in your body is that of numbness, cold fingers, etc., if it is hot, the sensation you would feel include, sweaty fingers, alertness, etc.

In both situations, your brain would be telling you different stories about how terrible the weather is, how much you should detest winter or summer, etc., these stories will make you feel worse. In extreme situations, it is best to stay with the sensation. The truth is that it is very difficult to stay with the sensation, it can however be practiced.

Here is the practice routine to follow, as recommended by *Ruby Usman:*

1. Find a comfortable spot to sit. It should be in a way where any part of your body can easily be reached by your arms.
2. The location does not really matter; it can be outdoors or indoor, what matters is that you are comfortable. Also, while silence is usually preferred, you can play cool relaxing songs too to get you in a relaxed mood.
3. After taking position, take a few deep breaths.
4. Now, you should start placing your hands on different parts of your part and feel the sensation. To do this, you can start from the top and then go down or you can do it vice versa.
5. As you place your hands on different parts of your body, you will start to feel the sensation. The next thing is to name that sensation. Whatever the sensation you feel, be it cold, warm, numb, relaxed, or even nothing, just allow yourself to feel it and name it.
6. As we have recommended earlier, that you should place your hands on different parts of your body, this part involves placing your hands on as many places as possible – everywhere that you can touch – including your genitals, back of the head, pelvic area, cheek, crown of the head, etc.

Take your time with this practice, it may take you about 15-20 minutes depending on how you practice it. When you are just starting, you may not feel anything, especially if you are not used to connecting your body sensations. However, as you start to feel it, your progress will be rapid. You can practice every day or as much as you like. Doing it every day is advisable because it will help you stay with the feelings when extreme feelings come at you.

The third and final step is to create a resources list. This is a list that you can easily go to when you want to feel better, and you need to give yourself more energy. For instance, when you feel sad or anxious, what are the things that make you feel better? What are the things you really enjoy doing? What makes you feel safer or calmer? All these are important because there would be dark periods when you will feel like giving up or abandoning your journey. During such periods, the resource list would come in handy.

A resources list consists of the following categories:

1. *Activities that you can do yourself*
   - Lightening a candle and then watching the flame
   - Take a walk in a quiet and natural place
   - Cry
   - Dance
   - Listen to music
   - Meditate

2. *Activities that can be done with friends*
   1. Talking about your pain and hurt with them
   2. Ask for support
   3. Getting hugs

3. *Activities that can be done with your romantic partner*
  - Go on a special date
  - Asking your loved one to hold your heart
  - Spending quality time with your partner

There is no rule or formula to this, it is just good to create a list and keep it close. The resource list could be all or any of the things listed above. There is nothing wrong with wanting to be reassured, being loved and being supported. It is important for you to inform your friends and loved ones beforehand, so that they can be sensitive to your needs.

Deepen Your Personal Tantric Practice

Tantra practice embodies love, Tantra itself is love. With the practice of Tantra, you can harness the energies around you and channel them towards spiritual enlightenment. The practice of Tantra reveals to us how we can balance and integrate our masculine and feminine energies, for us to feel whole again. With Tantra, one's understandings are revamped, and one begins to see the Divine and sacred in everything experienced and encountered.

The practice of Tantra brings more love and presence into your life. Here are some practices and exercises that may help you deepen your personal Tantric practice as a lover:

1. *Change of orientation:*
  When we talk about a change of orientation, I mean the practitioner having a change of perception and starting to see things the right way. People would normally refer to intercourse between partners as 'sex', while in Tantra, we regard it

as *love-making*. Love making goes beyond the stage of thrusting, it involves merging both energies, and the partners becoming one. For this reason, it is important to have a change in mentality. Making love is sacred and it involves rituals.

2. *Meditating and setting intentions before love making:*

It is important for partners to sit and meditate before engaging in sex, this should be done in some comfortable sitting positions with the partners facing each other. Doing this will help you call forth your highest selves, and it would help you offer your bodies to a higher power. I talked about setting an intention earlier while discussing how to heal sexual wounds, setting an intention will guide you through.

Meditating also will help you set the mood right, and it will help you understand the sacredness of sex. Setting intentions should be done together; you should be clear about the intentions you are setting, together and individually. You need to ask each other what you want to offer to the Divine through your love making.

3. *Make a commitment to be present:*

It is important for the two of you to make a commitment to be completely and truly present with each other. This will help you to create a pure and true atmosphere, it will help you both feel your energies and feed your energies. Often, people are too afraid to be completely open, to dig deep or to be vulnerable. With your partner, this should never be a challenge. In fact, doing this will help you improve your love making, and it will help you understand each other more.

While going through the process, you should ask about the stage your partner is at, this will help your love making. For instance, for a woman, if her yoni is not wet, it is definitely a sign that her a body is not ready to receive her partner. If this happens, you should make a conscious attempt to open yourself up, and remove all blockages that may be hindering you.

4. *Practice Tantric massage:*

Tantra massage allows you to worship the body of your partner; worshiping both the yoni and the lingam, as Tantra recommends. Practicing Tantra massage allows you to build intensity before love making, and it allows you to explore each other's body.

Tantra massage is the perfect preparation that you can enjoy for the act of love making. However, yoni and lingam massage are not compulsory part of Tantra massage; you may give your partner a Tantra massage without yoni or lingam massage.

5. *Learn control:*

Learning how to control is very important both in the acts to lead to love making and love making itself. Without the ability to control yourself, you will not be able to get maximum pleasure or give maximum pleasure to your partner. Learning control is very important, especially for men. It is important for men to learn how to hold their seed. Tantra encourages men to retain their seed, as this sends the energy back into the body upon reaching orgasm.

This allows the man to be energized, instead of being drained and this energy is then used for higher spiritual purposes. It also men become alive, focused and present after love making.

6. *Have no expectation:*

Often, when people make love, the expectation is to reach orgasm. Having this expectation does not create a deep intimacy for partners after love making. The goal or agenda should be to commit to freeing up energies within you merging them with your partner's. This will help you create an amazing bond with your partner, it will also help you reach climax easier.

Deepening your personal Tantric practice with your partner is very important when you are trying to develop both in your relationship and in your personal life. There is the need for you to continuously expand your understanding of Tantra, and to continue explore the paths to enlightenment that Tantra traches. Tantra offers the path to peace, love, healing, pleasure and most of all enlightenment.

CHAPTER 2

"When the breath wanders the mind also is unsteady. But when the breath is calmed the mind too will be still, and the yogi achieves long life. Therefore, one should learn to control the breath."

-Svatmarama, Hatha Yoga Pradipika

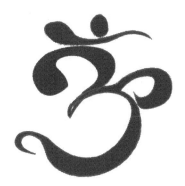

Building Trust with Sacred Touch

THE ROLE AND IMPORTANCE OF TOUCH IN A RELATIONSHIP cannot be overemphasized. Touch and communication are very important in keeping any relationship alive or in reviving a dead relationship. Touch is an essential part of Tantra Yoga, especially for intimate couples and to deepen the intimacy in their relationship. A lot of people, especially those who do practice Tantra, do not know this secret. When partners do not touch each other enough, they lose out of a lot of things, and it has the tendency of making either of them feel unwanted.

The human receptors have the inherent ability to sense touch and this helps us to connect with our partner and create a bond that is strong. The wonder and the knowledge of touching is not limited to Tantra, it is a universally open and is known to a lot of people, but practiced by very few. The practice of Tantra, however, can help you achieve intimacy through touching effectively and with more depth.

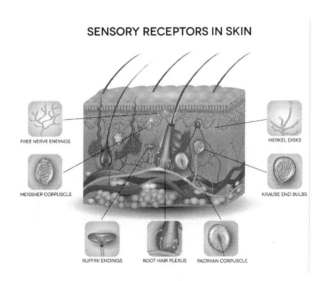

SENSORY RECEPTORS IN SKIN

FREE NERVE ENDINGS

MERKEL DISKS

MEISSNER CORPUSCLE

KRAUSE END BULBS

RUFFINI ENDINGS   ROOT HAIR PLEXUS   PACINIAN CORPUSCLE

Even though touch is a powerful tool in building relationships, it has destructive abilities too. Too many times, people get violated, and they get touched by strangers or even known people ways they do not like. This happens to people a lot, and it makes a lot of people shrink when they are touched; even when the person touching them is a trusted partner. It is therefore important for partners to be able to build trust with the way they touch each other. Touch does not always have to be sexual or for the purpose of love making, touching your partner gently and affectionately is important to building trust in a relationship.

The practice of touching to build a connection is very important to every relationship; learning it increases the chances of such a relationship surviving. The importance of touch is also very crucial in having good and thorough sexual experience with our partner.

The 21st century world could be a fast, tension-soaked, and crazily selfish one. We are always focused on achieving one target or another without a care as to what is happening to the other person. We have been completely bought over by the speck of setting and achieving goals that we have forgotten the goodness inherent in touching our partner.

Everything shouldn't be about you because the world doesn't revolve around you or your desires. When everybody sees the world the way you do then the issue of touch deprivation will worsen. We have to make the world and its people feel safe enough to allow others make contact with them. The best way you can help to reduce this touch dysfunction ravaging the world is by learning to touch and be touched without expectation or aim.

There's so much that the world can gain when people learn to hold, hug, and massage one another for the simple purpose of spreading goodness. A touch devoid of sexual motivation. A touch for the purpose of intimate connection.

Parents touch their children compassionately even when they are being reprimanded. A gentle touch will speak love to them as against spanking. Even when they need to be disciplined, do it with a gentle touch. Couples should never be tired of touching and massaging each other. Touch each other randomly. Let the other person know that he or she is valued, respected and worthy of sacred touch.

The practice of Tantra will teach all the above and more. The truth is that our survival on this earth as Divine beings is largely dependent on touch.

We live in a society where almost everything is about giving and receiving. The man wants to touch the woman as a means of arousing and leading her into sex just to satisfy his sexual urge. The woman too, when she's flooded with sexual energy, wants to touch her man and use him to satisfy and quench her sexual urge. We've gotten used to this act of getting what we want by either giving something little or nothing that we've forgotten how it feels to give for the simple pleasure of giving.

The same way the child needs the loving and caring touch of the mother is how partners need the loving touch of each other for a better love building experiences. Romantic touches don't have to end in clitoral or ejaculatory orgasms and doesn't have to be done for these reasons. When orgasm is the driving motive for engaging in touches then the best that we could do is the release of built up tension and as pleasurable as it might be it is nothing compared to the deeply satisfying experience of Tantric touch which grows love.

From the practice of Tantra, we are learning that touch can be so much more than the avenue to experience mutual masturbation. It can take on the path of increasing whole body arousal and building of trust between partners. When touch is viewed from the lens of Tantra, it begins as a conscious touch which stirs energy across the length and breadth of the body. This minute electric charges begin subtly, build up and continue to grow until the entirety of the body is reached. The pleasure waves that comes with this electronic waves helps to increase the body's happy hormones which will open up the heart and the free flow of sexual energy.

> The arms are our most obvious outlet for the display of love and the palms are the focal points. Tantric touches are not only a show of support and love for our partners but also that of healing of any disappointment, pain that the day's experience might have brought along.

Learning to touch the Tantric way helps in the building of trust. When a man or a woman understands that the touch from their partners is not for the purpose of intercourse for which they might not be ready for, it's easy for them to surrender their vulnerability both physically and spiritually and trust that the other person will keep to his or her word. When participating couples respect the "just touching" agreement between them and their partners, over time it helps to build trust and both of them will begin experience great touching experience together.

Apart from trust building, Tantric touch helps in the alleviation of debilitating patterns that may lead to emotional or sexual disease or dysfunction.

Practicing Sacred Touch

The first sense we develop as humans is the sense of touch because it allows us to feel pleasure and comfort, to connect with self, and to heal. Touch is the doorway through which the discovery of the true essence of our spiritual, sacred, and sexual being can be unraveled.

Why is Tantric Touch different from other forms of touch? It is sacred. *How is it sacred?*

Touch mean different things to different people. It may be a show of love, support, or affection. How we view this touch affects how it is handled. The sacredness of Tantric touch comes from the fact that it's a meaningful touch and isn't done to take advantage of a person as a way of getting what we want but as a way of reawakening our consciousness and unleashing our sexual energy. Tantric touch challenges how we view touch and teaches us that there's more to gain than *in-the-moment pleasure.*

The sacred touch of Tantra is a great way to reawaken your dormant sexual energy, reconnect with your deeper self, and heal wounds. It's also a wonderful way of discovering the joy inherent in receiving. Tantra brings about the merging of the body with the spirit through self-awareness.

Tantric touch, other than for it to be fully experienced, is without agenda. The aim isn't orgasm or performance even if the genitals are involved. The receiver together with the giver are fully aware of what's happening. They are allowed to go beyond the boundary of pleasure and also feel love, emotion, and every other aspect of their being. The more these thoughts saturate our body the more self-aware we become.

How does this work?

> Tantra believes that the man is not a solid being but rather a vibrating body of energy. This energy can also be in the form of sexual energy. Tantric touch helps in the activation of this energy and as it spreads through the body it feels like pleasure. This sexual energy passes between the body of the one receiving the touch and the one who is giving it so that none of the two feels like the receiver or giver.

In Tantric touch, there's no leash on the level of pleasure that we can feel and it doesn't have to reach a climax where it is completed with intercourse or orgasm. There's no withholding it and instead we surrender to it. We can feel pleasure to the maximum and every part of the body can be affected, not only the genitals.

Tantric touch is active and isn't passive for both the receiver and the giver. The recipient isn't just lying there receiving the touch. He or she is in the moment, and letting go of tension, resistance, negative thoughts and any other negativity capable of constricting the heart, body or mind.

The Art of Touch

The art of touching is an important part of Tantra massage and love making. As you must know, at this stage, the practice of Tantra is sacred and everything it teaches allows humans to access a level of enlightenment that is beyond the ordinary. Also, touch is a powerful and important form of communication; it transfers energy. In Tantra, emphasis is placed on the importance of touch in Divine union and connecting both bodies to the Divine.

Touch is scared, because of its sacredness, it is important for you to do some things before you touch your partner or before you start to establish a touch connection.

1.   *Be clear with yourself and ask yourself some important questions such as: is your energy pure?*
     If your energy is not clear, then that it is what you will be transferring to your partner. You need to know what you are taking to the table; did you have a stressful day or is there anything that disturbing your mind? All these things need to be cleared before you make an attempt to touch your partner; clear your energy field. We discussed the importance of being present earlier, these things are going to keep you from being present. Touches transfer energy, make sure you are transferring positive and pure energy.

     You have to make sure that your *higher-self* is present and totally in alignment with what you are doing. You need to ask yourself why you are doing it? Are you doing it because your partner wants you to, because you want to get money from or just because you want to have sex with someone? Touching is not meant to connect you and your partner on a physical level alone, it is meant to connect you on a deep spiritual level too. It is, therefore, very important for you to do it only when you connect with your partner beyond the physical.

2. *Stay out of your mind*

When contact is made with someone, a lot of things go through the mind. In fact, the mind will take you on several journeys, and this will not make you present in the moment. It is important for you to stay out of your mind, and be present not only physically but mentally and spiritually also. This is usually a very difficult thing to do, however, it can be achieved by allowing yourself to feel! Feel as your partner feels, feel their breath, feel their skin and the warmth of their body; get into your partner's passion and become one with them.

3. *Revere your partner*

People often make the mistake of thinking that they are with their body during love making. No, you with a temple, a sacred temple; revere it. Each person is a being that houses the Divine, therefore, you shouldn't treat them otherwise. When you are able to recognize the privilege, you have to access your partner's body, the process of making love with them becomes different.

When you are able to recognize this, you'll be full of nothing but worship for your partner. When touching your partner, you are not only worshiping the Divine in them, you are also worshiping the Divine through them.

4. *Open your eyes and make eye contact*

For a lot of people, closing their eyes or looking away during touching or full sexual intimacy is usually the best option for them. The reason for this is usually because they are afraid of true intimacy and how vulnerable they'd be. In Tantra, however, it is important to make eye contact with your partner.

Opening up and being vulnerable is not a bad thing, it is, in fact, vital in understanding each other. Making eye contact will make you see beyond the physical eyes of your partner, it will help you see into the deep recesses of their soul. When touching your partner, especially in the case of a massage, stop intermittently to look into each other's eyes. In the case of making love, it is not enough to be in your partner physically, you should be in each other through your eyes too.

5. *Learn to touch*

Based on unfortunate experiences that people have had, especially women, they find it hard to trust people's touch or even feel comfortable when they are touched. Learning to touch your partner will help them trust you, and it will make them feel more present when you touch them. For people who have experienced sexual trauma, they find it hard to stay out of their minds when touched, they may start to think of their past experience. However, when you are able to lead them to trust your touch, it becomes healing for them.

Touch doesn't always have to lead to sex, touching can be done to your friend or anyone. Therefore, you should learn to touch and be touched without the expectation of anything to happen after. This can be practiced with your friends, even of the same sex. You should learn to touch your partner without any sexual undertone.

Tantric Massage Techniques

There are many ways in Tantra to achieve a great sexual experience with multiple orgasms for anyone who opens his or her heart to it. A Tantra massage is an effective way of building up sexual tension between partners and get intense pleasure, sometimes, without any penetration involved at all.

Tantra massage is a good way to communicate through touch, and have a mutually sexually satisfying experience. There is no certification needed to give a Tantric massage to your partner, all that is needed is loving guidance and focus.

To start this process, it is necessary that your mood is perfect for this kind of experience. In setting the mood right, you have to make the environment perfect for it. Things like dimming the light, lightning candles and burning some incense can work in setting the mood right. It is best to use oil for Tantra massages, it could be scented mineral oil, essential oil, massage oil, etc.

When you are about to start, start with the back side. Pour the oil you have prepared for the occasion into your hand, about two tablespoons should do the magic while starting. Rub the oil on your two palms, then place your hands on the backside of your partner and move your hands up to the neck and around the shoulders of your partner, caressing her back. Do this repeatedly, moving your hand back, all the way down to the buttocks, over the buttocks and the rosebud.

The next is the hand slide. This involves placing your hands parallel to each other and sliding the, down each side of your partner's spine. Doing this, you massage all the way down to the lower back and over the buttocks. This should be done repeatedly too, at least for about six times. The next after this is the pull up, and this involves alternating between hands, as you stroke the side of your partner's body.

Kneading is another amazing Tantra massage technique. This involves squeezing your lover's back and buttocks between your thumb and fingers with one hand first, and then the other hand; this should be done in a flowing motion. After this, slide your hands to another side of the back and repeat the process until every area of the back has been covered.

Feather stroke involves caressing the neck of your partner, including the shoulders, arms, back and buttocks. This is usually done with the fingertips, applying light feather strokes for about five minutes. You can gently scratch your partner with your fingernails also, if they are well trimmed. Another way to apply this technique is for women who have long hair to use it on their partner – a man with a long hair can do this too. To make use of your hair, gently use it to caress your partner's body. It is a very erotic massage that will arouse them. It should be noted, however, that doing this will definitely get oil into your hair, it should be done if only you are comfortable with that.

After you have worked on the other part of the body, you can then move on to foot caress. To give your partner a foot caress, you will need to apply all the other techniques you have used on the body here. You may start with the kneading stroke, and then follow it with the feather stroke. Don't attempt to do both legs at the same time, do it one leg at a time. The feet are sexually sensitive, so it is good to pay attention to them. Slide down the bottom of each foot with your palm, do this back and forth repeatedly and gently. Finally, rotate the toes gently, clockwise and vice versa.

After massaging the back of your partner thoroughly, it is time to turn them over, and concentrate on the front side. It is time to concentrate on the stomach and chest region. Repeat the same process from the back, however, with more details on certain areas. For instance, kneading can be done on the male chest, but feather stroke is a more appropriate technique for a woman, especially around the breasts. Concentrate on the nipples because they are a great source of pleasure, both for the man and the woman.

When these techniques are applied appropriately, it would create a new level of sensual connection between you and your partner.

A Tantric massage involves mindfulness and loving touches. There's no standard way of practicing Tantric massage and there is no predetermined outcome. This type of massage is not limited to specific parts of the body, the entire body participates and erogenous zones can also not be left out.

Being an energetic massage, Tantra places great attention on sexual energy. The aim of Tantric massage is to intimately connect the one who gives the massage to the one who receives it. This reception can be physically, emotionally, mentally, or otherwise. This massage moves the person in the direction of an ecstatic state of consciousness or awareness, leading to a great mental, physical, mental wellbeing.

It's a wonderful avenue of relieving tension, improving blood flow, moving energy all over the body, and sexually arousing your partner. It helps couples to attain mutual satisfaction and increased intimacy and connection. With a society, full of people who have, one way or another, being starved of touch, Tantric massage provides the avenue to end this starvation.

Everybody can give a Tantric massage and you don't have to be a certified therapist to do so, all that's required is for you to follow some guidelines. Since there's no standard techniques for a Tantric massage, you can always find various Tantric massage techniques so long as they have two basic ingredients of a loving touch and attention. The core of Tantric massage is the heart or intention with which the massage is done.

Steps of a Tantric Massage Technique

Begin by taking a shower or bath to relax yourself and prepare the body for the massage. This is more like a purification ritual. Play some music and preferably something you enjoy without words. Use some essential oils to fire things up and cover yourself in something like a towel or a sarong. Here, the body is gently tapped, rubbed and kneaded as a way of relaxing it.

1. *Introductory Massage and Vertical Positioning*
    As you begin the massage, the giver places him or herself in a vertical position in relation to the receiver, as a sign of respect to him or her and as a way of bringing harmony between you. The giver begins to massage your body and you can only lie there and enjoy it. You begin to see your senses awaken,

your attention sharpening, and waves of pleasure passing through your whole body.

2. *More Massage*

    As this masseuse or masseur continue to touch your head, hands, trunk and feet, you begin to relax while all your tension and stress take flight. With essential oils and a hot towel, your body massaged to a state of intense body sensations and deep relaxation. Using feathers, furs, and soft objects, the already sensitized body is tenderly massaged, causing a rain of excitement to flow through the body. At this stage, hot lava stones can be used as a means of warming the body.

3. *Intimate massage*

    This stage of massage is a slow one and involves the intimate parts. As your Yoni or Lingam is being carefully and tenderly massaged, you can experience the flow of energy from your intimate parts to your head, and passing through your spine.

    Now you can begin to practice breathing as he or she joins and mirrors you in the breathing, your awakened energy spreading all around your body. Your body is now completely saturated with a self-healing and self-nurturing energy, and you're deeply relaxed.

Relaxation Rituals

Any Tantric massage isn't complete without the relaxation rituals. Tantric massage and relaxation rituals are combined to produce a wonderful therapy of complete and deep relaxation.

Knowing the importance of a relaxed body to the whole massage process, every Tantric massage begins with a relaxed and gentle rubbing, tapping, or kneading of the body. This initial relaxation massage is better carried out in a personalized manner for the recipient where his or her specific needs are taken into consideration. This general practice normally begins with long gentle strokes, as a means of relaxing the body.

The relaxation ritual that is been talked about here is different from the deeper Tantric relaxation rituals done at the end of the whole Tantric massage, and as pleasing as the above relaxation practice is it isn't the same with the final relaxation ritual.

The Tantric massage practice is separated into three distinct stages. The first stage is a relaxation ritual. This takes between 5 or 10 minutes and the aim of this part of the Tantric massage is the relaxation of the recipient and preparation of the body for the massage. This is sometimes referred to as the purification ritual.

The second stage is the massage proper and has an average duration of 30 minutes or more. This stage of the Tantric massage begins after the initial 5 or 10 minutes' relaxation rituals. This is the part where the body is seriously massaged and tended to. This stage of the Tantric massage is what will give continuity to the awakening of sensations and new energies, bringing about deep relaxation.

Tantric relaxation is conducted after the Tantric massage as taken place. For this relaxation ritual, the recipient lies on a futon (*a couch or bed can also be used in the absence of a futon*) and with eyes closed, allows the experience to sink in. The giver caresses the recipient and directs the energy till it goes around the body and then settles.

Tantric relaxation ritual has its own advantages. It lowers stress and anxiety, helps to stimulate blood and lymphatic flow, disperses tension points, and leads to new relaxation levels.

The relaxation part of Tantric massage is quite different from normal relaxation massage. In Tantric relaxation, you're full of energy and even go straight to work because you are fully alert and conscious while normal relaxation massage causes the recipient to feel sleepy.

If by now you haven't figured it out it, let me once again reinforce it that touch is a very important part of our humanity. Whether you're aware of it or not, something is being communicated through touch.

Practicing the art of selfless, intentional, inspiring, and meaningful Tantra touch will open up wonderful doors for you and others. You will experience peaceful and relaxed body. Calmness and relaxation beyond the ordinary.

Tantra massage opens you up to the wonderful experience of a freely flowing, unobstructed, revitalizing, and inspiring life energy which will cause your emotional injuries and blockages to disappear. You will go through physical, mental, and emotional release of these blockades.

Tantra doesn't only open your body it also opens your heart, making you more aware, more loving, more sensitive. You are able to experience life better and see it from an enlightened standpoint. You're are on your way to being joyful, blissful, and ecstatic.

CHAPTER 3

"A rose is an opportunity for beauty to happen.
The physical body is an opportunity for love to happen.
Tantra is an opportunity for Godliness to manifest through us,
so that we, as limited beings, can share in the
ecstasy of the Universe."

~ Osho

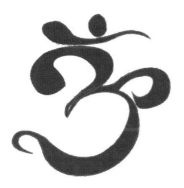

Merging
Sexual Energy

IT HAS BEEN EXPLAINED EARLIER THAT LOVE MAKING or sexual intercourse is not just the act of physical penetration of man into woman, in Tantra, it is far more than that. Sexual intimacy connects the spirit and it merges the soul. When people engage in the act of love making, energies are released by the two people and these energies can be merged to form a strong spiritual bond between the two.

Sexuality is sacred in Tantra, though for many Westerners, this seems to be an absurd statement; to declare that sexual intimacy is sacred is to declare that there is more to it than just than just thrusting and orgasm. The truth is, there is indeed more to it than just thrusting and orgasm.

We live in a society where we've been made to believe that sex is a way to release tension built up in the body. We spend sexual energy in engaging in some minutes of sweaty exercise so as to release this tension and in the end, we only end up losing more energy following the release.

The appropriate response to being flooded with sexual energy isn't to just release it. Sex can be so much more than the avenue to release tension. It can be spiritual and a path towards higher level of consciousness. Sex can be an opportunity for the merging of the masculine and feminine energy.

Sexual energy which is one of the highest form of energy and when it's correctly channeled can bring us to state of cosmic connection to the source of life itself. This happens when this energy is harnessed and directed from the pelvic area up the body to the head, where the mind is activated

Yoni Massage: A Woman's Journey

The term "Yoni" is Sanskrit for vagina which is also known as "sacred cave." We cannot disparage or disregard the role played by the sexual organs in our emotional, physical and spiritual health because it is paramount. It is so important that when these organs experience blockages because of toxins, the ability to create and spread this energy, which can also be called Prana; chi; or life force, around the body is greatly reduced. The ability of the body to carry out its self-healing activity is dependent on these organs.

A woman's vagina and sexual energy are her power sources. These power sources are imbued with the power to liberate the individual and provide her with life-shaping power.

Your state of consciousness is reflected on your body. Your life's experiences particularly in the case of unresolved issues are conspicuously written on your body. These unresolved traumas can cause energetic blockages of these power sources in various parts of the body including the reproductive organs. If these traumas are not dealt with and its attendant constrictions released, they will show eventually as physical ailments such as low libido, sexual pain, numbness, menstrual and menopausal struggles, difficulty in orgasm, lack of sexual lubrication, etc.

These ailments didn't just appear from nowhere; they are the results of the things going on in your body. Your reproductive organs act as emotional and traumatic stores of all that happens in your relationships and sex life and when they are saturated with blocked energy, there can actually be a disconnect between you and your reproductive organs. So, when these things appear as physical ailments understand that they are telling you something and it's that they need healing, love, and attention.

At birth, your Yoni was filled with pleasurable and positive cells but when issues like traumas, accidents, surgery, etc., came, this once positive force became a negative one. The emotions attached to these negative activities become stored around these sexual organs, disconnecting you from them. The organs became numb and painful and unable to feel pleasure or orgasms.

Yoni massage provide you with the opportunity to heal. When you are healed, you will experience a magnetic yoni which will cause good things to be drawn to you; you will be led towards good decisions and great things; you will be full of orgasms, particularly the ones originating from your vagina; you will experience a better life; you will resurge great ideas in your consciousness.

Female ejaculation which is referred to as *Amrita* in Sanskrit can be experienced during Yoni massage. This type of ejaculation helps to eliminate negative emotions so that the pelvic area is free of them, therefore making sexual energy positive, freeing, and open. This creates space for the growth of positive sexual energy. Also, Yoni massage provides you the chance to experience body shivering, shaking, and spasms referred to as *Kundalini Awakening*. This helps to unblock the blocked or negative energies round the entire body so that the body can experience full and total body orgasm. This experience can last for many minutes and can even be as much as hours.

Yoni massage provides you with a great opportunity to heal, awaken, and supercharge your reproductive organs, especially your vagina.

In Tantra Yoga, the female body is expected to be approached with reverence and adoration. Specifically, the vagina, it is a part of the woman body that Tantra Yogis approach with a sense of worship. As we all know, sexual organs play a lot of important roles in our physical, emotional and spiritual wellbeing. The woman's vagina is her gateway to receiving and releasing sexual energy, however, there are many ways this may not be achieved. Briefly, I will take you through the processes of a yoni massage.

Yoni massage is becoming a very popular term, and it is gaining a lot of mainstream attention in the West. But what in itself is yoni or a yoni massage? What do you stand to gain by surrendering yourself to it?

When translated into English, yoni loosely translates to "a sacred place". This meaning succinctly captures the whole point about the sacredness of sexual intimacy. For a practitioner of Tantra, the yoni is to be approached from a place of total respect and love – from loving reverence.

In contrary to a lot of Western philosophies and ideologies that only celebrates the male penis, and see the vagina as a tool only for the pleasure of the man, as where Tantra respects the vagina. To a large extent, the reason why there are more female victims of sexual wounds is because the female vagina is seen as merely being a tool for the satisfaction of men, and this makes a lot of men feel entitled. In Tantra, however, the practice of yoni massage is meant to truly and genuinely honor the woman and her body. It is meant to give true and selfless pleasure and to explore the sacredness of woman sexuality.

A lot of women rarely experience orgasm, other people who, only experience one orgasm in the process of love making. *Yoni massage is not about having a single orgasm, it goes beyond this to the level of trying to feel more and more pleasure that will result in multiple orgasms.* The yoni is meant to be worshiped throughout this massage, and the process is expected to give the woman multiple orgasms throughout the massage.

The interesting thing about a yoni massage is that it can be done with or without a partner. A lot of the ability of a woman achieving orgasm has been placed on the ability of the partner, but with yoni massage, multiple orgasms can be achieved without a partner. It can also be done individually or as a buildup – foreplay – to the act of love making. Also, this massage is very good for women who have never had orgasm.

Yoni massage is a journey towards understanding your body. For those who have suffered from sexual wounds in the past, it is not only a journey to understanding your body, it is also a journey to *reclaiming your body and your sexuality.* As explained, yoni massage is about worshiping the vagina, so the process is not supposed to be rushed at all, it is supposed to give you time to slowly explore your body in very sensual ways you have never experienced before. It is a journey because it helps release emotions and energy that have been stuck in the womb, it not only does this, it also continues to help you discover new areas in your vagina that feel good.

To start exploring your body or to help your partner start exploring her body, here some processes that can be followed for maximum results:

1. **Set the scene:**

    It is important when you start, especially if it is your first time, to start with an open mind and an open heart. Do not attempt for any reason to judge yourself or your body. To start, find a comfortable place to lie on your back, with a pillow under your hips. Put your knees up and your feet on the ground parallel to your body. One essential thing you need for this is your massage oil you find comfortable to use.

2. **Connect to your breath:**

    Earlier, I spoke about the importance of breathing in Tantra, however, this is addressed in the form of partners participating the practice together. In this case, you are not expected to breathe together with your partner, you are expected to practice this alone. For yoni massage, you are also going to practice bliss breath.

    To start, you will have to constrict the back of your throat and inhale. When you do this, you should hear a whispering sound, after this you should then exhale and release the whispering sound again. Continue with this routine of slow, open mouthed and deep breaths with audible sounds. Doing this will ground you in your body and keep you out of your head. Furthermore, it will help to spread the orgasmic energy all through your entire body. When you practice this right, it can help you move the energy from your yoni to other parts of your body.

3. **Warm up:**

    Foreplay is not only important in the process of love making, warming up the body is very important prior to a yoni massage. Body massage or a Tantric breast massage can be very useful in warming up the body for the practice of yoni massage. When you warm up your body, you get relaxed, and you gradually and slowly build up arousal.

The best place to start is usually the belly. The belly is often overlooked when people talk about pleasuring the woman's body, however, it is a very important center for pleasure, as it has many nerve endings. You should gently massage the rib cage, between the breasts and the lower abdomen.

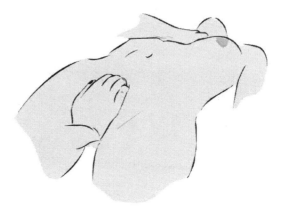

Gradually, your body will start to respond. When this begins to happen, you should slowly circle the breasts before doing same for the areola. While circling the breasts, do not leave out the nipple. When your body, or the body of your partner, starts to respond more to the massage, you can then start to tease the nipples. You should try to alternate between circling the breasts and light pinching.

At this stage, it is expected that the body should be charged and properly warmed up for the yoni massage. You can then start the yoni massage properly. Here are five techniques to use of yoni massage.

1. **_Circling:_**

This can be done by using the tip of your finger to circle the tip of the clitoris for the stimulation of arousal. The circle you make can vary from small circles to bigger ones, and the pressure can always be alternated from light to heavy, for maximum pleasure.

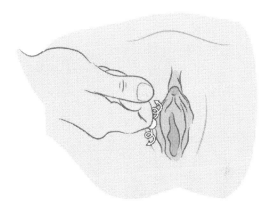

2. **_Pushing and pulling:_**

What you do when you are trying to apply this technique is to push down on the clitoris, and then make a small push and pull stroke. After this, you can slide your finger down the shaft of the clitoris. Slide your finger down on both sides of the clitoris, but do not forget that some women are more sensitive on different parts of the clitoris than the other. You should also bear in mind the reaction of your partner at each stage. If you are doing it yourself, you should take note of your body's reaction at every stage as well.

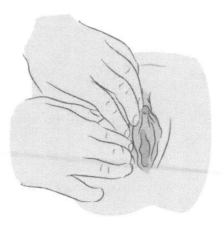

3. *Tugging and rolling:*

The clitoris can be tugged by pulling it gently away from the body by grasping at the sides and tugging it back and forth. After doing this, you can decide to move lower and tug the sides of the lips. To roll the clitoris, hold it firmly and roll it between the thumb and the index finger.

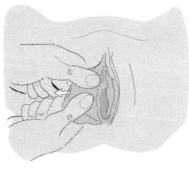

4. *Tapping:*

The tapping technique is done just as it sounds. Using your fingers – one or more, start to tap the clitoris in different pace and rhythms; tape it slowly and then quickly, and then switch paces at intervals. Doing this will help you know what the body responds to the most.

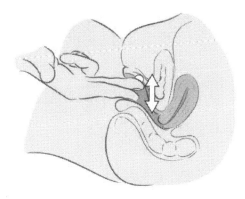

5.   *G-Spot Massage:*

G-spot is a word that even a novice in the process of sexual intimacy have heard about. The problem is, people only talk about it, they are not equipped to explore it. With yoni massage, every part of the vagina is explored and worshiped.

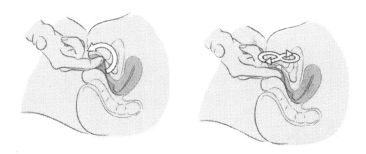

To discover the G-spot, curve your first two fingers to make the shape of the letter C, and then slide the fingers into vagina. When your fingers are in, still curved, feel for a soft, spongy piece of skin behind the clitoris, that is the G-spot. You can massage it gently with the two fingers, and then alternate the strokes between fast and slow. While doing this, you can tease the clitoris as well, to give maximum pleasure.

These five techniques are not meant to done one after the other, they can mixed-up for maximum experience. Of course, it is good to start in that order, but when the body is fully charged, you can tease the nipples while you stimulate the G-spot. In fact, the fun and the special thing about yoni massage is that it is meant to help you explore your vagina and worship it, it is not meant to give you a manual for doing this.

Honoring the Lingam: Your Pillar of Light

Tantra is concerned with moving and heightening the body's sexual energy for pleasure, healing, and spiritual awakening. The practice of lingam massage is another way of making this possible. The lingam is a pathway to free the soul. *What exactly is a Lingam?*

The word *'Lingam'* is Sanskrit for penis, and means *"wand of light"* in literal terms. The practice of lingam worship and honoring is commonly carried out in several spiritual traditions and involves a worshipper and the one whose lingam is worshipped. In the ancient practice of lingam worship, the worshipper does it unconditionally. Just like the vagina, the penis is a sacred tool that can be used to release energy. It is meant to be loved and respected just like the vagina. It is important for a man to come to the full understanding of his body works and help your partner understand your body too.

The lingam symbolizes generative energy in Sanskrit. It isn't about bringing a man to the state of orgasm (*even though this is a welcomed side attraction*) but about bringing him to a state of peaceful relaxation and higher consciousness where he receives good doses of pleasure. This practice is a way to build intimacy when it's done between partners.

When skillfully carried out, the recipient can fully relax and build up sexual energy which will be channeled around his body. This art is capable of awakening great moments of pleasure in the recipient in ways he has never experienced before and this experience is always earth-shattering and soul-touching.

In lingam worship, the penis is massaged in a way the receiver releases bottled-up stress as it relates to issues of relationships, self-esteem, sexuality, etc. The aim is for him to come out feeling deeply relaxed and with heightened sensitivity.

The principle behind lingam massage is energy movement. The body's sexual energy which might be lying dormant is energized and caused to move and thereby causing increased pleasure, healing, and heightened spiritual awareness and consciousness.

This energy is activated and channeled round the whole body causing it to awaken magical and pleasurable moments, the type the body has never experienced. These awakened moments will then lead to feelings of unmeasurable ecstasy, touching your soul in ways that words cannot describe. The receiver is deeply relieved of any stress and is able to relax after the process.

To be clear, a lingam massage should not be mistaken for the typical erotic massage which leads to happy endings. The aim of lingam worship isn't ejaculation, as a matter of fact, the aim of lingam massage or worship isn't to ejaculate.

The lingam has a way of reprogramming the recipient's sexual DNA and turning him to the sexual being that he was created to be.

Like I said earlier, the goal of a lingam massage isn't ejaculation, but a means of activating and putting the body's energy into good use. That's why the lingam challenges the receiver to refrain from ejaculation so as to retain this energy, even when engaging in sex. When you retain this energy through non-ejaculation, you can then direct the power and the seed known as *Ojas* towards that which is Divine. Therefore, it is always said that Tantra, no matter how connected to sexuality it is, the ultimate aim is enlightenment, happiness, and inner peace.

By honoring the lingam, this is a way of respecting the Yang in him. When you honor your man this way, his unconscious extra power is stimulated. Began by planting three kisses on the tip of his lingam as a show of respect and blessing. Think about what it takes for a man to give up control of his body to another person. This ability to relinquish his penis should be greeted with honor and demands his penis be treated with utmost reverence and care.

A lingam massage provides the recipient with benefits like enhanced ejaculation control, intense sexual pleasure, increased blood circulation to the reproductive organ, enhanced sensitivity, cure of premature ejaculation, improved sexual stamina, alleviation, and relieves stress, pain, and depression.

There are challenges with lingam massage, however, with guidance, these challenges can be resolved. The first challenge is that a lot of men find it hard to open up and free their minds to receive pleasure. To be able to do this fully, you need to be able free up your mind and feel a lot of emotions and sensations which lead to vulnerability. A lot of men do not want to feel vulnerable, they want to feel safe, and this may be a big challenge at the end of the day for a lot of men. However, the vulnerability you feel while practicing lingam massage is not meant to make you feel insecure, it is meant to set you free.

The second challenge is that a lot of women do not feel comfortable with handling their partner's penis. This could be so for many reasons which are peculiar to each person. To be able to overcome this challenge, it is important for the woman to take time to reflect on the problems, the negative impressions they may have about the penis. Some of these negative impressions may not be based on personal experiences, but impressions gotten from the society and social norms.

The lingam massage is, in two ways, just like the yoni massage. First is for the men to learn, as this will empower them to be able to practice edging themselves, through self-massage. The second is for the partner, the partner would be the one helping the man through this practice. When done with a partner, it can either be done independently or as a foreplay to love making.

The practice of Tantra helps partners connect with each other on a personal level. It helps the partners understand each other's bodies and know how to pleasure each other. Furthermore, it is important for partners to be able to connect with each other's universal sexual chi, and of the ways to build this connection is through lingam massage.

The whole concept of lingam massage may sound strange, but broken down, a lot of people will say it is just a fancy word for foreplay. However, a lingam massage is done with respect and reverence. It is done with more thoughtfulness and the desire to help your partner achieve great pleasure. Lingam massage is not just about stroking and orgasm, it is about paying attention to every detail and every part of the lingam and using some advance techniques to get the desired result.

The man's penis carries a lot of sexual energy, learning to stimulate the penis and circulate the sexual energy is very important and powerful. This practice is done to honor the man, and it is expected to be all about him for that period. The man's penis is very crucial to having a sacred sex and it should be approached as a very sacred place.

Just like the goal with yoni massage, lingam massage is not just about getting an orgasm, it is about working with your partner to achieve more pleasure that will lead to waves of multiple orgasms.

To get started with a lingam massage, you first need to create an atmosphere that is perfect for the practice. It is important to create safe and sacred space where the massage can be done. Creating a space does not mean you go to a sacred place, it means you make the space you have sacred and perfect for the practice.

You need to create the right temperature that will make your partner, a warm temperature will help your partner relax. Having the right light and sound is also a very good way to set the mood for the massage. Finally, you need the right massage oil for this practice, the same thing applies for lingam massage as with yoni massage. When you have been able to get the environment set for the massage, you can then delve into it. Here are the steps and techniques to follow for an effective lingam massage.

1. **Get him relaxed:**

    Before you start the massage, you need to get your partner relaxed and comfortable. This can be done by having him lie on his back in a very comfortable place; pillows can be used to make him more comfortable. The knees of your partner can be bent, while his legs are spread apart, to make it convenient for you to reach every part of his genitals. You can sit between his legs or beside him.

2. **Breathe:**

    Again, the bliss breath is necessary here. Breathing is very important in Tantra, in fact, it is what separates Tantra sex from regular sex. It is important to breathe the bliss breath while giving your partner lingam massage, this will help you receive his energy of arousal and pleasure when you inhale and then send him loving energy when you exhale. The breathing goes both ways. Breathing while performing this massage is very important because it helps you understand his feelings more, and it makes you empathetic to his thoughts and feelings. Not only this, it will also help in heightening the sexual understanding between you, it will help you become aware of what your partner wants even without communicating about it.

Breathing together, at the same pace and with the same rhythm, will put you both at ease. It is important for you to keep reminding your partner to keep breathing deeply and feel relaxed while you perform the massage.

3.   *Connect:*

It is important for the two of you to connect on the same level. This can be done by placing a hand on the chest of your partner – on his heart, and the other hand on his genitals. It is important for you to breathe together here too, and look into each other's eyes for a few minutes. This physical connection will help you connect on a much deeper spiritual level.

4.   *Lubricate and massage around the genitals:*

It is now time for you to apply the massage oil. Rub the oil on your hand and then start by sliding your hands up and down around his thighs, and gently stroking his groins. Move to his perineum and stroke it gently also. Then move to his testicles, and start massaging them gently and slowly. If your fingernails are not too sharp, you can use them gently on his testicles, teasing them gently and slowly.

It is important to communicate with your partner while the massage is going on, this will allow you to understand how he likes what you are doing. This is important because men react to touch differently, and getting his reaction would help you know the next step to take.

5.   *Massage the penis:*

If he likes what you have been doing so far, it is time for you to move to the penis. Start by massaging the shaft of the penis, alternate between grips, switching from light to hard grips. You should also try to alternate between stroke movements, switching between up and down movements to twisting movement. Also, alternate between hands, change from left hand to right hand, and from one hand to two hands. Furthermore, do not keep it at a single pace, pressure or rhythm change between these things to give your partner a better experience.

Here are some ways you can alternate between strokes:

- Use both hands to hold the penis in the same direction, with the fingers pointing the same way.
- You can use one hand in holding the penis, facing one way, and the use the other facing the other way.
- Also, you can hold the base of the penis with one hand, and use the other hand to stroke up the shaft, all the way to the head. When you get to the head, corkscrew your hand off the head.
- Use both hands to slide up and down at the same time

There are many other ways focus, but the important thing is not to let him climax, you should try to keep him at the edge. To know if he is close to orgasm, you need to be able to pay attention to his breathing, body language and movement, and the way he his moaning. When you see that he is at the edge, pull him back by slowing down and calming him by reminding him to breathe.

6.   *Stimulate the sacred spot:*
One way to achieve great pleasure is to stimulate the sacred spot. A lot of people may be wondering that what and where

exactly is the sacred spot? The sacred spot can be found between the bladder and the penis, the walnut-sized gland located between the two. Specifically, it is the prostate. The sacred spot is very pleasurable for men, and you should learn to stimulate it properly for your partner.

The sacred spot can be stimulated either internally or externally. When stimulated internally, a finger or two are inserted into the anus to stimulate the prostate, or by using a prostate massage sex toy. When done externally, the outside of prostate is massaged without penetration.

For a man who is inexperienced with prostate massage, it is usually advisable to start externally. You can subsequently graduate to internal stimulation. To massage it externally, locate the sacred spot by looking for an indentation that is about the size of a pea and a walnut, just midway between the testicles and the anus. Push this indentation inward gently. It is important to be slow and gentle with your pressure. You can keep pushing in and out gently, or use a circular massage movement. Use plenty oil to help with lubrication.

If you man is comfortable, you can then take it internally by stimulating the sacred spot. Stimulating the prostrate internally involves penetrating the anus with your fingers or with a massage sex toy, therefore, you need the explicit consent of your partner. A lot of men may not be interested in having their anus penetrated, however, if he is interested, you can then take it to the next level. Start by loosening his anus with massage oil. Massage the exterior of the anus first, do this with your fingers in slow and gentle movements.

Before you insert your finger, make sure you apply enough oil to both your hands and his anus. Also, it is important for you to make sure your nails are smooth and well cut. Insert the tip of one finger first, it is advisable to use the little finger first. Use this to loosen him up by wiggling the finger around, back and forth his anus. When the anus is loosened, you can then insert your one or two fingers deeper to locate the prostate. Once you locate the prostate, start caressing it with your fingers.

To end the massage, you can make him climax with an ejaculation, or extend it to intercourse. At the end of the day, both of you would have experienced intense pleasure and deep connection.

Full Body Orgasm

Statistics show that around 90 percent of men experience orgasm during sex while only a meager 25 percent of women do. Despite these poor statistics, it's still possible for people to have not only multiple orgasms but full body orgasms. *How?*

The ancient practice of Tantra tells us that our body can be connected to the Universe on a cosmic level. The connecting vehicle is the sexual energy which resides in the reproductive organs and energy centers.

Apart from teaching us how to rediscover our body and that of our partner, Tantra also teaches us how to channel this energy away from the genitals, up above and to the head. When this sexual energy gets to the head, your body is made to vibrate at a cosmic level and this vibration brings about a full body orgasm.

When the sexual energy is awakened, and channeled to up the spine to the head from the genitals, a blissful release of this energy is experienced all around the body's system. When this happens, you will feel like a surge of electricity is passing through your body from the toes of your feet to the hair on your head. This experience is possible for both the make and the female.

Getting to this stage takes practice but the benefits you will enjoy as you take this journey will bring about great and dramatic changes in your body and relationship.

As you can see from the beginning of this topic, the problem isn't about whether the men and women reach orgasms or not but about the frequency and what it takes to get to the orgasmic level. So how can we, both male and female, experience full body orgasm?

We do not truly understand how powerful our sexual energy is and as a society we've been programmed to repress this wonderful energy in our genitals and only release them during clitoral orgasm for females and ejaculatory orgasm for males. Traditionally, when we are sexually stimulated to the point of arousal, we somehow tense our body, constrict it, and even hold our breath. This self-imposed tension and holding or constriction of breath locks this arousal in the genital region and prevent it from travelling all through the body leading to a localized and genital based type of orgasm. This experience becomes a release-type of orgasm and no matter how nice this experience may feel, it's nothing compared to the experience of a full body orgasm.

As a result, the Tantra practice focuses on body relaxation because it will prevent the practice of holding your tension in your body as doing so will prevent you from the ecstatic experience that the full body orgasm can provide. Also in Tantric practice, emphasis is placed on free, deep breathing. Your breath is the vehicle that carries this sexual energy round the body. So, what else can we benefit from full body orgasm?

It's a Tantric belief that the sexual energy is very potent and capable of energizing, healing, and rejuvenating the body. It also helps to clear the mind and inspire creative intuition. This explains why men and women who have learned to channel their sexual energy are more energized and seldom feel sleepy during the day. They also have their minds flooded with profound clarity and amazing creativity.

Men and women, but mostly the men, often feel exhausted after ejaculatory or a clitoral release, and more likely to doze off after the experience especially when it occurs at night. These and other sexual effects can be greatly minimizer if sexual energy is channel through the whole body. It's even better when this energy is retained in the body through what is known as non-ejaculatory orgasm.

Both sexes can and should have not only multi-orgasmic experiences but also full body orgasm. If you truly desire an energetic, deeply satisfying, multi-orgasmic, full-body, and deeply nurturing ecstatic states, you should consider towing the Tantric path.

A lot of Tantra masters and adherents believe that humans possess sexual energy and when this energy is blocked or constricted for any reason, the person whether male or female experiences issues that may lead to some physical ailments like lack of orgasm, premature ejaculation, depression, etc...

Shiva is worshiped in the form of Lingam and while Shakti is worshipped in the form of Yoni. A lingam is a vertical, rounded column, representing the male creative force and the infinite, indescribable nature of God. Yoni which represents the female creative power and energy. Together they represent the union of organs, and the totality of creation.

Through the practice of Tantra, these energies can be correctly channeled to improve relationships and sex life. It can also lead to the lifting of restrictions in the body. This will cause the recipient to be more awake, have increased sensitivity, enjoy heightened sexual vigor and improved health.

"The body can become a vehicle to that which is beyond body, and sex energy can become a spiritual force."

~ Osho

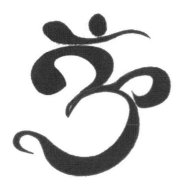

Part 2: Tantric Movement & Energy

CHAPTER 4

"Breath-centered asana practice and Pranayama are among the greatest gifts from the Yoga tradition to help us maintain our physiological and metabolic health and well-being, balance our emotions, and clarify our minds."

~ *Gary Kraftsow*

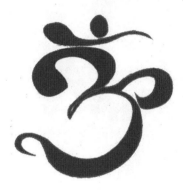

Yoga & Tantra Rituals

TANTRIC PRACTICES ARE WAYS IN WHICH WE CAN integrate and merge life into spirituality, and it helps us live in peace and harmony both with ourselves and those around us. Essentially, Tantra rituals utilize the elements of the Universe through the process of action. For Tantra yogis, it is believed that everything in the whole Universe is a field of energy, be it a living thing or not. And these energies can be tapped into and harnessed to free the mind and achieve enlightenment.

Tantra is a practice that involves a lot of rituals. However, the purpose of these rituals and the practices is to help focus the mind and deepen the devotion of the Tantra yogi. The rituals are merely a means through which a Tantra practitioner can attain a higher state of consciousness. According to *Ashely Thirleby*, the author of *Tantra: The Key to Sexual Powers*, she stated that "the rituals make it possible to enjoy sex more often, for longer periods of greater pleasure than you have ever known before. And the more frequently you have sex, the more quickly and powerfully your sexual energy will regenerate itself."

The primary aim of Yoga is the awakening and balancing of the body's subtle energies. The body is made up of seven fundamental energy centers. The practice of a Yoga pose (*Asana*), is a means through which the body's energy centers which are also known as Chakras can be connected to the equivalent subtle energies of the Universe.

Asana is a tuning system or one that brings into resonance through which the two systems of the Universe or macrocosm is linked to the human body or microcosm by mentally evoking the desired effect. This is possible because they both have the same vibration frequency.

Asana practice is not only physical in operation, it is also mental. When taking a Yoga pose, you evoke the desired effect by simply thinking about something like pure love or happiness or peace and concentrating on your heart chakra. This is the secret of a Yoga pose, and when correctly carried out it can bring about a resonance between the limitless macrocosmic sphere of love and the body's heart chakra, and by transferring virtually unending quantities of loving energy from the heart.

Whatever exists in the macrocosm also exists in our microcosm and this what is known as the law of correspondence. While the subtle forces in the microcosm are often dormant and exist in a state of potentiality, the macrocosm are fully energized with unlimited power. So for a person who has the possibility of experiencing pure endless love may actually not experience it because there's no resonance between the person's love-energy and that of the macrocosm. The practice of Yoga helps to bring about this resonance.

Yoga can help the practitioner cultivate love, not only for yourself but also for others. So, all you have to do when you get on that Yoga mat is to open up your heart. The advantages of doing this goes far beyond the physical, it permeates all levels of your being. Yoga postures can help invite more love into your life by increasing your resiliency, and elevating your mental clarity and consciousness. So get busy!

Asanas of Love for Kundalini Arousal

Kundalini is an energy that manifests consciousness when it gets unleashed. According to Hindu philosophy, *Kundalini* is that Divine energy that is located at the base of the spine. It is a vital energy that lies dormant until it is called upon and unleashed. It is often represented as a snake curled up, lying dormant. Kundalini exists in all of us, but it is not a physical force that can be observed or detected by an MRI scan.

Kundalini awakening is when this Divine energy is called upon and unleased. The best way to achieve kundalini awakening is through the practice of Yoga, Breathwork, and combining visualizations and stillness. When the awakening is attained, the practitioner achieves a level of understanding about and spirituality of life. Awakening kundalini can also happen as a result of hallucinogenic, deep sexual experiences, trauma etc., and if not under the guidance of an experienced teacher, it can lead to psychosis. Once you experience a kundalini awakening, life and existence will never appear to you the same again. With appropriate guidance, it can help you free up blockages and achieve true purification.

If we allow it, there is a wonderful flow of energy, love, and light, waiting to explode and swell from within your heart center. We can open it up by practicing kindness, joy, and acceptance. We must also embrace all emotions, and recognize every single one of them as beautiful.

Here are some poses that are common to Kundalini awakening:

Easy Pose (Sukasana)

With this pose, you are expected to cross the legs at the ankles, then you press the lower spine forward to keep the back straight. Make sure the ankles are comfortably pressed on the floor. It can be done by placing both feet comfortably on the floor too.

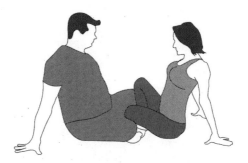

Perfect Pose (Siddhasana)

For this pose, the right heel presses against the perineum, sole against the left thigh, and the left heel is placed on the right heel and it is made to press the body above the genitals. Also, the toes are tucked into the space between the right calf and thigh. You should make sure that your kneels are on the ground, with one heel directly above the other.

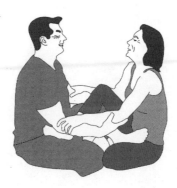

Lotus pose (Padmasana)

Here the left foot is lifted on top of the upper right thigh and the right foot is placed on the left thigh, both are then placed as close to the body as possible.

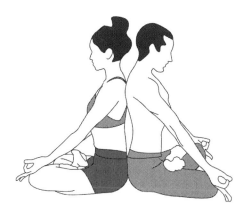

Celibate pose (Virasana)

The feet are placed wide apart, and the practitioner then kneels and sit between the feet. This posture is believed to channel sexual energy up the spine.

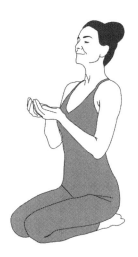

Matsyasana (Fish Pose)

How To Do:

• Fully extend your legs and relax them

• Roll to each side while hiding your arms and your palms facing the floor, under your body.

• Push your elbows down while inhaling and produce a beautiful letter "C" using your back.

• Close your eyes and drop the topmost part of your head to the matter.

• Point your toes down and slightly engage your thighs.

• Inhale deeply into your ribs and picture your heart explode and swell with absolute bliss.

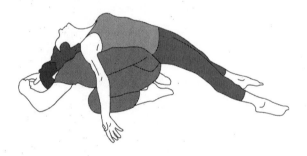

Supta Virasana (Reclining Hero Pose)

How To Do:

• Lean backwards slowly into the mat, and ease yourself down onto the upper part of your back. Protect your knees, and if need be, use a blanket or a bolster to support your lower back.

• Draw out your arms above your head, allowing your palms to make contact and your skin kissing the ground.

• Inhale deeply into your belly and your chest.

• Bring your hands to your heart center and move your fingers out and apart from each other in the form of a blossoming flower.

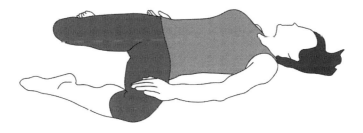

Ustrasana (Camel Pose)

How To Do:

• Straighten your spine, sit lightly on your knees, and raise your arms above your head

• Bring back your arms slowly behind you as you fold backwards and try to touch your heels.

• Form a subtle arch in your spine by grabbing, holding, and dropping the crown of your head in the direction of the floor.

• Picture your breath growing deep, and your ribs opening.

• Breathe in fully and push out all the air in your belly and then your chest.

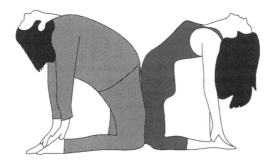

As stated earlier, love making is one of the ways to achieve kundalini awakening. Love making in Tantra is a way of connecting to the spiritual and reflecting on the Divine. That is why it is not something you do with just anybody, it is to be done with someone with a connection with on an emotional level, and someone who shares your thirst for the Divine.

Partner Yoga Sequences: (*side by side*)

It is an amazing feeling when you practice Tantra Yoga sequences, but it is even more amazing, when it is done side by side with your partner, it makes the two of you connect on a much deeper level both energetically and physically.

Apart from the fact that Tantra Yoga helps you build spiritual connection, the quality time you spend together is very important, so you should try to focus on the connection with your partner and enjoy the presence of each other.

Yoga is a means of unifying. A steady Yoga practice helps to inspire communication and love between participating partners. The partner Yoga practice isn't meant to be a competition but a means of supporting one another. It will definitely bring laughs and it may even bring tears, but above everything else, it will foster a feeling of connection and create a better way with which the partner's body can better communicate with each other.

There are certain things that must be put into consideration before you engage in this practice:

- Be sure to warm up and relax after it's done,
- Don't engage in anything that may cause your partner to be uncomfortable, and
- Before trying Yoga on your own you must try to learn from a certified Yoga instructor.

Here are some simple sequences that partners can try:

Partner Tree Pose

This pose helps to develop focus and confidence, and improves balance. It also strengthens the thighs, core, spine and ankles while bringing the partners together the more. It further stretches the inner thighs and groin.

How To Do:

• Stand close to each other and, while placing them in front of your heart, draw your hands into prayer pose.

• Find your weight on the leg closest to that of your partner, lift the outside foot, and place it on your thigh or calf.

• When your feet are steady in this tree pose, try to connect to your partner

• To reach your palms together, draw up your inside arms

• At the medial line between the two of your bodies, draw together your outside hands and join them in creating prayer hands.

• After a while, you can slowly come out of this pose, get your balance, and bring back the outside foot to the floor.

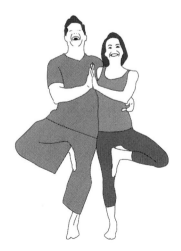

Partner Warrior 2 Pose

This pose, part from its interpersonal benefits, also helps to improve strength, balance, and stamina.

There are many warrior poses, and each of them can be done in Tantra. For this pose, it is important to always maintain eye contact with your partner to deepen your connection. Stand with toes of your right feet touching that of your partner, then move your left feet backwards to about three feet, moving your toes out at a 45-degree angle. After this, you should then bend your front knees and straighten your spines. Finally, drop your shoulders back, square your hips towards each other and attempt to raise both of your hands above your head. This can be done repeatedly by switching sides.

How To Do:
- Facing the same forward direction, partner A should stand sideways with partner B.
- Together touch the insides of your feet.
- Reach with your inside hand, and put it on the upper arm of your partner.
- Turn your outside foot out and by 90 degrees, turn it away from your partner, and raise your outside arm so it is parallel to the floor.
- Breathe in deeply and, as you force out this air, let your back hand slides along the arm of your partner toward his/her wrist as you bend your outside leg to a right angle.
- For like 6 to 8 breaths, take the final posture while firmly gripping the wrist of your partner.
- When done, release your hands, straighten your legs, and switch places.
- Repeat on the other side.

Seated Twist

This is also called the seated spinal twist, and it is a way to warm the spine and use each other to deepen your flexibility. To start, sit in a comfortable position with your knees touching each other, then sit up straight, with your chest pushed slightly forward. The shoulders should be pushed back and the chin pointed slightly down.

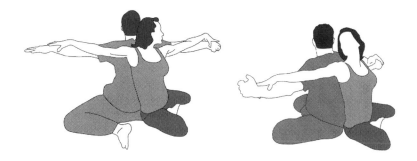

After this, place your left arm behind your back, and extend the right out. This should be done by the two of you. When you do this right, your partners left hand will reach out your right hand, and your left hand will reach out to your partners right; grasp the hands as they reach out to you. The result of this would be a twisted body by the two of you. When your hands are connected, try to twist as far as you and your partner can get comfortable with. To twist, you need to communicate constantly with your partner. Maintain the pose for a while before switching sides and repeating the pose.

Yab Yum

This is a pose that will help you align your energy with that of your partner. To start, have a partner sit cross-legged on a mat, then have the other partner sit on the thighs of the partner and cross their ankles behind the back of their partner. Try to be aligned with each other and to keep straight; this can be done with the use of the abdominal low back muscles. Align your foreheads, let them touch each other gently, then try breathing deeply and slowly together at the same pace.

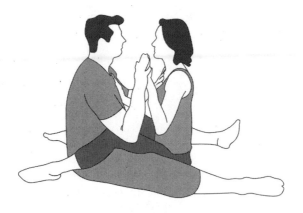

Heart-to-Heart & Hand-to-Heart

This is a very simple pose that can help partners achieve deep connection in silence. With this pose, there is no need for any communication whatsoever. One partner lies down on their back, and the other partner lies next to you, with the second partner slightly above. It involves looking deeply into your partner's eyes, and placing the palm of your hand over your partner's heart. Looking into each other's eyes will help you see further into your partner, and placing your hand on each other's chest will help you feel each other's heartbeat. You can try to breathe together slowly and harmoniously. After a while, you can switch places with your partner.

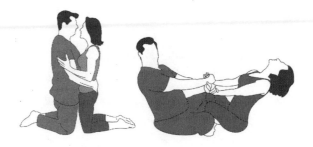

Legs up the wall

This is a pose that can be performed with your partner in child's pose, and it allows the two of you to rest at once. It is a restorative pose.

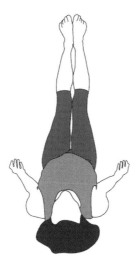

To start, have your partner kneel, their head touching the ground, and their hands stretched out and relaxed. After your partner has gotten into position, sit on the hips of your partner, facing away from their head. Then, lay back on your partner, with your spine made to curve of their own spine. The final stage is to raise your legs into the air. After completing this, the next thing is to switch positions with your partner.

Shared Savasana Pose

As the standard ultimate relaxation position in nearly all Yoga practices, this pose not only helps to relax the body, it also helps to maintain breathing and tactile connection between partners.

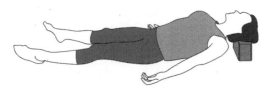

How To Do:

- Begin by lying down side by side with your partner

- While in this position, make sure there's enough room between the both of you to hold hands and also rest your arms.

- While tuning into the sound of your partner's breath, synchronize your breathing as you hold hands and relax together.

Partner Yoga Practices: *(for each other)*

1. Twisting and Turning

This pose adds energy and vigor to your body, strengthens and stretches your body, and releases all its locked tensions. It also helps to inculcate, in you and your partner, a sense of playfulness and fun.

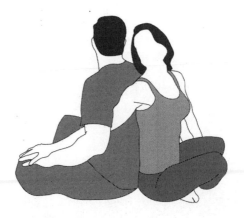

How to Do:

• Take a Sukhasana pose while your backs are facing each other.

• While feeling connected to your partner, breathe in and put your arms over your head.

• Breathe out and twist to the right, while placing your right palm on the left knee of your partner and your left palm on his/her right thigh.

• Let your partner turn the same way and place his/her palms in the same manner.

• When you both come into position, hold the pose for a couple of breaths.

• Breathe out, and return to your initial position.

• Repeat this by turning to the opposite side.

2. Boat Each Other

This pose gives you plenty time, ambience, and space to reconnect with your partner while also strengthening your core and energizing your body.

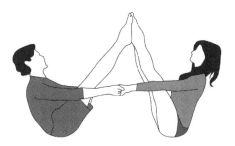

How to Do:

• Sit down facing the opposite direction with your knees bent, and toes touching one another.

• Reach out to the wrists of your partner and hold them.

• Get your knees nearer to your chest while lifting your feet, let your partner do the same.

• Straighten your back and heave your chest up while taking support from your hold of the wrist of your partner.

• Slowly and gently lift up your legs. When your partner takes the same position, touch the soles of your feet to those of your partner.

• Take a few breaths while staying in this pose. Then release gently from the pose

3. Build A Heart

This pose helps to open up your shoulders and chest, and increase your spine's flexibility. It will also help to make you feel light in the heart.

How to Do:

• With your backs facing one another, stand straight.

• Hold both your hands tightly together, arch your back backward, and raise your heads upwards.

• Fall forward you and your partner, and use the support of your tightly held hands to allow the back of both your feet touch one another.

• This pose will form a heart-shaped symbol.

• Keep this pose for a few breaths and release it in a balanced manner so you do not trip and fall.

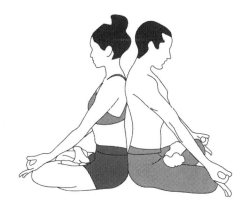

Yoga can provide the practitioner with a rewarding experience especially when it's done with a partner. Partner Yoga can add variety to an otherwise boring routine and is a very good way to practice Yoga from another practitioner.

There's a lot to gain from the unique practice of Yoga and Tantra. You can employ it to improve your connection. The practice breeds understanding, and brings about deep and loving relationships.

CHAPTER 5

"For breath is life, so if you breathe well
you will live long on earth."

~ *Sanskrit Proverb*

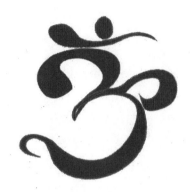

Working
with Chakras

WE ARE SURROUNDED BY ENERGY IN THE ENTIRE UNIVERSE, our body itself, is a bundle of energy. In Tantra, any object whether living or not is seen as an energy carrying object, and they can all be channeled to achieve a higher level of awareness. Is essence, there are seven major centers of energy that move permeating us.

Chakra is a Sanskrit world that can be translated to mean *wheel*. Chakra refers to the seven main energy vortexes that make up our consciousness and energy mapping system. The work of chakras is to function as pumps that regulate the flow of energy in a clockwise direction. The chakras determine a lot of things about our perception of reality and how we choose to react to situations in our life.

You may be wondering why the word is called a wheel, it is so because the life force that moves inside everyone spins and rotates. The spinning energy, starting from the base of the spine, all the way to the top of the head. In the body of a healthy and balanced individual, the seven chakras provide exactly the right quantity of energy to every part of the person's body, mind and spirit. However, if one of the chakras spins is too open, spins too fast, or it is too closed, the individual's health may suffer.

When you have good knowledge about the chakras, you will become more in tune with the energy cycles of your body.

The human body, according to the Yogic tradition, the chakras have huge roles to play with how we breathe, live, and express ourselves. Healthy chakras translate to healthy mind, body, and soul. Unhealthy, blocked or badly functioning chakras can lead to illness.

We may not be aware of this but every one of us has received this; criticisms, insults, unsavory remarks, enables us to close our chakra. When this happens, our creative ability or expression is limited and we find it difficult to speak for ourselves in truth.

No doubt life can be frustrating sometimes but you can experience inner peace and have healthier behavior patterns if you learn to work with your chakras. Chakras are very effective when it comes to providing you with new insights, innovative ideas, and a rewarding lifestyle when you choose to open their doors. You can work in one of the most pressure-soaked, tension-filled, and highly stressful environment and still be able to feel relaxed and brush away all the negative energy that comes with the job.

Open chakra doors are an opportunity for more psychic, energetic, and spiritual capacity while closed ones brings limitations with them. With rightly flowing chakras you can better manage your well-being, exude more confidence and communicate your hopes, dreams, and thoughts more eloquently. It will be like you have a stress-proof layer, and you will be able to function in a more focused and relaxed manner. When you're working with your chakras your natural immunity will greatly increase and you will be better suited to handle stress.

The thing is, we might not be able to control our environment and how people interact with us, but we can control how we react to our environment and the people that we interact with. The practice of chakra tuning will help infuse you with inner poise and balance. When this practice is bolstered with a healthy diet and positive activities, the best of yourself will come out to the world.

The Chakras Resolve in Tantra

It is important to get hold of your body and release all blocked energies for both your physical health and for spiritual awakening. Understanding how your chakras work and how to keep the energy flowing freely is very important. Even though the chakras are not physical, however, each of the seven primary chakras is connected with one of the seven endocrine glands, they also connected with a group of nerves plexus. As a result of its connection with the plexus, each chakra is connected with particular parts of the body and performs particular function in the body controlled by the plexus or the endocrine gland which it is associated with.

I've said this before, but for the purpose of emphasis, let me repeat myself: *the whole of the Universe is a sea of energy of which our body is a member. Ancient cultures have since recognized this life force as present in all living things.*

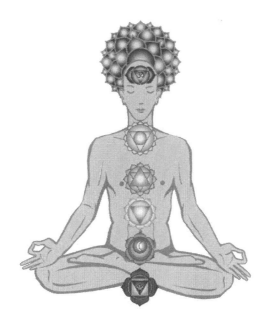

The word Chakra is of Sanskrit origin and it means disk or wheel. This life force or *Prana* rotates or spins around permeating the body. This is why Chakra is known as the spinning wheel of energy or light. It is the center of energy inside of us and this energy emanate to other parts of the body to help us function at optimal levels.

For a healthy and balanced person, these seven chakra energy centers feed the body with and distribute the correct amount of energy to all parts of the body, mind, and spirit. When these centers are working correctly, the whole of the body experiences harmony and health but if there's a problem with any of them causing them to be too open or too close or spin too slowly or too quickly, the individual's health will suffer.

By understanding how these chakras work and how you can work with them, you can become more in tune with your body's natural energy cycles. You can also learn to harmonize your emotional, physical, and spiritual imbalances.

When learning to work with the chakras, it's generally advised to begin the opening of the chakras from the lower ones before moving up. Open the root chakra first then move on to the sacral chakra. From sacral to move to navel, heart, and then third eye. Ending with the crown chakra.

Here are the seven chakras:

1.   The Root Chakra - Muladhara:

The Sanskrit name for this chakra is *Muladhara*, this comes from two words; *Mula*, which means *root*, and *Dhara*, which means *support*.

This means that root chakra plays the role of connecting all your energy with the Earth, a practice which we call grounding.

This chakra is located at the base of the spine at the tailbone in the back and the pubic region in the front. It is associated with the basic need of safety, security and survival. When this chakra is blocked, issues like low self-esteem, fear, anxiety, frustration, etc. may occur. It is also common to have problems with obesity, anorexia nervosa, and knee troubles, leading to feelings of helplessness, unworthiness and unhappiness with your physical body. Extreme blockage may lead to depression. The root body parts are; hips, legs, lower back and sexual organs. Sexual organs are the hormonal glands associated with it.

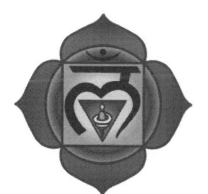

The color red is associated with it, and it is overactive when your survival instincts are super charged, even when there is no apparent threat. This is associated with the need to survive and restlessness.

The root chakra is underactive when you feel sluggish, lazy, tired and you are afraid of change. This chakra gives you the energy to take care of your survival needs first, and this should be utilized appropriately. You can then calm this chakra by focusing on your connection to spirit. It is important for you to find time to align yourself with the root by meditating, and performing acts of kindness and compassion.

2. *Sacral Chakra - Svadhisthana:*

Sacral is the second chakra, and it is located just the bellow the bellow the belly button, and it is rooted into the spine. It is from the Sanskrit word *Svadhishana*, and it translates to, "the place of self". As the interpretation states, it is the chakra that houses the creative energy, and your identity. The sacral is the place that hold the basic need for sexuality, creativity, self-worth, and intuition.

The color associated with this chakra is orange, and the body parts associated with it are; kidney, sexual organs, bladder, and large intestine. If this chakra is blocked, an individual may feel manipulative, obsession with thoughts of sex and may feel emotionally explosive. The secret to balancing the second chakra is to enjoy life modestly; live your life to the fullest joyfully, try to draw energy away from selfish pleasure into your heart.

3. *The Solar Plexus - Manipura:*

The Sanskrit name for this Chakra is *Manipura*, and it translates to "lustrous gem". It covers the area between the navel and the breast-bone. It is center of personal power, and also the place of impulses, anger, passion, etc. When this chakra is in balance, an individual feels a sense of wisdom, personal power and decisiveness.

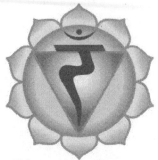

The color for this chakra is yellow, and it is associated with the stomach, liver, gall bladder, small intestine and pancreas. When this chakra is out of a place, an individual may feel depressed, confused, lack of confidence, feel that others are trying to control their life. When it is overactive, an individual may lack empathy or compassion, have anger issues, feel the need to control others in situations.

When it is balanced, however, the person will feel cheerfulness, enjoy taking on new challenges, has strong self-respect, and a huge sense of personal power.

4.   *Heart - Anahata:*

This chakra is located behind the breast bone, and it is referred to as the heart chakra. The Sanskrit name is *Anahata*, it translates to 'unhurt' or 'unstruck'. It is the seat of love, kindness and compassion. This is easy because the general symbol of love and compassion is the heart. This chakra connects the triad of the body, mind and the spirit. Also, it drives the openness of someone to love, and to receive love.

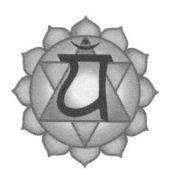

The color for the heart chakra is green, and it is associated with the following body parts, heart, lungs, circulatory system, upper back and shoulders. When this chakra is overactive, you may feel jealousy, possessiveness, overly sacrificing, and poor boundaries. When it is underactive, however, a person may feel antisocial, cold, loneliness, or withdrawn. When it is balanced, it comes with feeling of peace, empathy, love, and compassion.

5.   Throat - Vishuddha:

The Sanskrit name for this is *Vishuddha*, it translates to *very pure*. It is located in the "**V**" of the collarbone at the lower neck. This chakra is the center of communication, sound, and the expression of creativity through thought, speech and writing; it gives your personal truth a voice. The human throat is the place where anger is stored and also the location to let go of. Also, the possibility for change, transformation and healing are all located in this chakra.

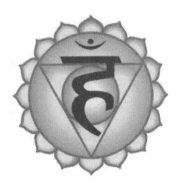

The color blue is used to represent it, and the body parts for it are; throat, ears, neck, thyroid gland and teeth. When it is balanced, musical and artistic inspiration may come, good oratory and great communication, also it helps to be a good listener. When it is out of harmony, however, an individual may feel like holding back, find it hard to express their thoughts, feel timid and weak.

6.   The Third Eye - Ajna:

The Third Eye is the sixth chakra, and its Sanskrit name is *Ajna*. Ajna can be translated to mean *beyond wisdom* or *to perceive*. This chakra allows you to access information beyond the material world. It is located just above the physical eyes, on the center of the forehead. It is the chakra for higher intuition and psychic abilities. It is also the center for energies of spirit and light. Through the power of this chakra, you can receive guidance, and tune into your higher self; it is helps with the purification of negative tendencies and selfish attitudes.

The color for this chakra is indigo, and the body part associated with it are, the eyes, face, lymphatic system, brain and endocrine system. When this chakra is out of place, an individual may either be afraid of success or be egoistical, feel non-assertive, lack imagination, denial, difficulty concentrating, and have nightmares. When it is balanced, people feel like they are the captain of their own life, have good memory, and great imagination.

7.   Crown - Sahaswara:

The Sanskrit name for this is *Sahaswara*, it translates to *thousand-pedaled* or *thousand-fold*. It is referred to as the *crown*, and it is located behind the top of the skull. This is the chakra of enlightenment and spiritual connection to the higher self and the Divine.

This chakra is probably the hardest to explain of all the chakras, however, it is best understood as the center of enlight-enment, spirituality, dynamic thought and Divine energy.

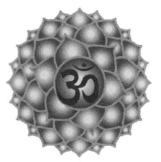

Achieving a balanced crown chakra could be perceived as difficult, because it can be compared to achiev-ing nirvana; it is the stage of direct access to the unconscious and the subconscious. Success in balancing the seventh chakra will make oth-er chakras fall in place. When this chakra is blocked, there may be a constant sense of frustration, destructive feeling, confusion, spiritual cynicism and lack of spark of joy. The color for this is violet.

It's not enough to understand that the body can sometimes experience energy blockages and constrictions, what's more important is learning how to resolve these blocks and setting the chakras free. This gist is that if you're in an emotional funk or are feeling less energetic and creative, there's a possibility that you have a clogged or blocked chakra. What exactly causes these blockages of chakras?

The chakras are the reservoirs of all the bad and good thoughts, actions, and actions that we've ever gotten involved in all our lives. While the good thoughts and actions will and has always brought us good memories and feelings of joy and happiness, the negative ones will only cause us to be sad, guilty and traumatized. As a way of escape, we try to repress the negative memories and thoughts and by so doing cause our chakras to shut down. This affects our posture, breathing, metabolism, and emotional state leading to pain, disease, and suffering which are all a product of that repression.

Another cause of chakra blockage stems from the inability of your mind or masculine side and your intuitive or feminine side to work together in balance and harmony. This disharmony can prevent the free flow of your life force.

The following are effective ways to resolve these blockages:

Forgiveness:

No matter how hard we try to deny it, the truth is that our past has a big role to play in our lives and they have a way if playing repeatedly in our subconscious mind especially when they negative. You may not even be aware that they're affecting your life, and it's only by accepting what has happened and feeling those emotions that we have fought hard to repress can we be whole again.

Forgiveness takes away the hold of these emotions so that we do not have to constantly relive them again and again, even when new events trigger them.

Yoga Practice:

Kundalini Yoga and Yoga poses like the cobra, camel, fish, and child's pose are a particularly effective way of releasing these energies. Stretching and movement helps to push this energy through the chakras away from where they are being constricted.

Physical Exercise:

Physical activities involving the exertion of force can help to move this energy. Walking barefoot, pelvic thrusts, dancing, writing, talking, eye exercise, and cardiovascular exercises are important for unblocking the chakras.

Spiritual Practice:

Apart from physical exercise, the practice of spiritual exercise like self-reflection, meditation, and contemplation is also a good means of removing these blockages.

Heat:

Heat helps to relax the muscles thereby allowing the negativity that's preventing the flow of the chakras to get out of the body. This heat can come in the form of vigorous movement, sauna, whirlpool, and any other heat source.

Nutrition:

The consumption of healthy red foods such as tomatoes, berries, beets, and apples; orange foods such as carrots, melons, oranges, or mangoes; yellow foods such as bananas, turmeric, ginger, pineapple, and corn; green foods such as avocado, broccoli, and leafy greens such as spinach or kale; blue foods such as blueberries, dragon fruit, currants, and kelp; and indigo foods such as purple kale, blackberries, and grapes can help to resolve blocked energy.

Chakras in Harmony

It is important to aim at achieving a balanced and harmonious flow of the seven chakras. When all the chakras are aligned, you are aiming towards a peaceful life. To be able to align your chakras, you need to first know the chakras that are out of balance, and that is why the knowledge of the seven chakras is very important. In reality, it is very hard to detect imbalance, however, it is good for you to be aware of your body and learn its signals and clues.

When you are aware of your body, it is easier for you to observe changes in the balance of your chakras. The best way to balance your chakras is through constant meditation and connecting your mind to the Divine.

Balance is a dynamic state, it's not static. When our body is constantly moving, we're oscillating between imbalance and balance, between harmony and disharmony. It all begins with awareness.

Awareness opens you up to understanding the clues and signals that your body gives. The more sensitive to your body, you can listen to the hints and instructions that it gives.

It's a fact that we're living in a fast-paced world with everybody always on the move. As we push ourselves to adapt to the fast nature of things we sometimes forget to take notice of how this creates imbalance and disharmony in us.

If we can learn how, it's quite possible to live and enjoy each day as it comes instead of being rattled and emotionally strangled by what our past was and what our future may likely be. This worry and the stress that comes with it will only make things worse because it will block our energy centers thereby affecting their functionality. When the flow of this energy reaches these points, it becomes stuck and cannot flow.

The products of a freely flowing and unrestricted energy or life force can be seen in the happy, good, ecstatic, and relaxed feeling of people who have learned to harmonize them. Anxiety, depression, and stress are some of the pointers to the imbalance, depletion and disharmony of this energy. As time goes on the individuals overall being becomes affected by this.

None of the different chakras in the body works independent of one another. Each one of them is a subset of the body's energy system. They all are part of a whole. The full functioning of each of the chakras is dependent on the full engagement of the others. Each chakra plays specific roles in the balancing of some aspects of our emotional, physical, mental, and spiritual life. So, the body is whole and healthy when each chakra plays its part.

It's a known fact that a lot of things starting from emotional, physical, and environmental this can affect our chakras, and when it does our energy becomes trapped or constricted. To deal with this block, you must find a way to remove this blockage and keep the energy moving. Doing this will restore our emotional, mental, spiritual, and physical equilibrium.

There are specific methods that can be taken to bring the body's chakras to the state of balance and harmony with one another. This process is a simple one and involves a simple meditation which will take you through each of your chakra. *The Zen and Vipassana Meditations are very effective at bringing you to a state where all your chakras exist in harmony with one another.*

Chakra Partner Practices

Relationships and Chakras are connected in an intrinsic way and the incorporation of some chakra practices has a way of strengthening relationships not only with oneself but also with his or her partner!

Awareness and intention has great roles to play when it comes to the success of relationships which is why a relationship connected to chakra is bound to experience deep connection, consciousness and intimacy.

Partners can engage in the following practices as a way of improving their relationships:

The Root Chakra Partner Practice:

This helps in the strengthening of the foundation of relationships. Practice this by sitting with your partner, shutting your eyes while holding hands. In this position, *focus on your root chakra by thinking about ways to better nurture your relationships and make your partner feel more secure in the relationship.* Share your idea with your partner after opening your eyes.

The Sacral Chakra Partner Practice:

Engage in this practice sitting with your partner, *closing your eyes, and visualizing your sacral chakra. During your practice, see yourself in the position of someone who's totally in harmony of his or her relationship.* Feel free to soak in the pleasure and wellbeing of this control that you have over your relationship. Share this feeling with your partner and display some level of affection towards him or her.

The Solar Plexus Chakra Practice:

Take a sitting position with your partner while enjoying a cup of tea together. Practice channeling your caring, respectful, loving, and strong energy. Each of you should then pick a conflict particularly a recent one and discuss it in a loving way. Sweeten the discussion with questions like, *"Do you feel different now that we have discussed this issue?" "Do you feel like this conflict has been resolved?" "Is there any other thing that you would like me to do concerning this conflict?"*

The Heart Chakra Practice:

Take a position where both of you are sitting close together with the palm of one hand on your heart and the other on your partner's heart. *While maintaining this position, speak to; what are the things that you love about your partner.* Take turns exploring this from a safe space maintaining eye contact and hands-to-heart.

The Throat Chakra Practice:

This practice involves the visualization of the color blue while sitting with your partner. Demonstrate your love towards one another with a touch, a notion, or a smile (*not words*). Each of you should then use words to communicate a thought that shows adoration for one another's unique personality.

The Third Eye Chakra Practice:

This practice is about clearing the path for openness in your relationship and it starts with you focusing between your eyes while sitting with him or her, visualizing the color indigo. *You can enjoy the practice by lovingly asking yourselves ways to improve openness in your relationship.* When you're done, let your partner know your thoughts about it.

The Crown Chakra Practice:

This practice is about seeking wisdom from your inner-guru and asking for clarity regarding your life goals, dreams, and deepening your relationships. *Close your eyes and focus on your crown chakra while sitting close to your partner. Even if you already know, still ask your partner what his or her goals are and how you can be of help towards its co-realization.*

Life is in a state of dynamic equilibrium and is not static. What this means is that all of what makes up our Universe and vibrate at a certain frequency. This means that our body is an ocean of vibration just as light and sound is not solid matter. Things are visible only because they vibrate a low frequency while the ones vibrating at exponentially high frequency cannot be perceived by the ordinary eyes.

As we have learned from the ancient Vedic history and culture of Hindu yogis, energy courses through our body via the specific channels. This energy through the specific centers for the spreading of this energy even beyond our physical sense or perception.

Each one of these centers vibrate at defined frequencies and has relations to specific emotional and physiological issues, organs and glands of the body, as well as colors and food.

This vital life force becomes stuck or restricted when something blocks their path causing them not to function properly. The result of blockages in these chakras will cause the body to fall into imbalance and disharmony and this will show outwards as illness and diseases in relationship, body, and mind.

By practicing forgiveness, meditation, visualization, Yoga postures and breathwork, good nutrition and some physical body exercise, we can learn to unblock these chakras and allow them course freely through our body.

CHAPTER 6

Feelings come and go like clouds in a windy sky.
Conscious breathing is my anchor.

~Thích Nhất Hạnh

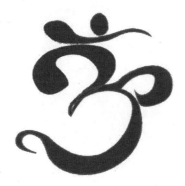

Breath & Stillness

PRANA IS THE SANSKRIT WORD FOR VITAL FORCE AND
this vitality is swept in by breath. This life force enters the body via
breath and sustains our life from one moment to another moment. As
this air finds its way to the body, the inner world becomes connected

to the outer world. The regulation of this life force via Pranayama provides a means for us to engage in free and conscious breathing. This type of breathing inspires us to connect with our environment and feel at ease with it. The more we engage in this, the more tranquility we experience, just the same way as the breath.

The idea of world peace is a noble one but what we must understand is that this world peace that we seek for must start from within. The peace must begin from within us. This inner peace and stillness can be received through our breath. A deep connection exists between breath and the mind and the mind can attain the state of tranquility, steadiness or stillness by conscious, deep, and free breathing.

Through Pranayama, the mind can become focused, peaceful, and still. Pranayama brings the mind to a state of stillness by the practice of exhaling the breath, suspending this breathe, and inhaling this suspended breath. This brings the mind into resting in a state free of thoughts, a state of complete stillness.

Our fast-paced world, one where you are only believed to be working when you're moving and you receive the label of lazy when you're still and quiet. The buzz and noise of this world has robbed us of what it means to be still. We no longer value being still, breathing or acknowledging this breathe leaving and entering our nostrils.

If we allow it, stillness can become a powerfully transformative action. It can help us in quieting the noise of the world and can teach us to recede from its buzz. The peace that we so dearly crave for on the outside can be achieved by peace on the inside.

The Power of Prana

Breathing and stillness are very important in Tantra. Breathing is a vital part of meditating and connecting to the Divine. A chaotic mind or a disorganized one cannot meditate, neither can it be consciously connected to the Divine. In order to be able to harness your energy, you need to gain mastery over your breath.

While making love with your partner, the role of breathing connects the forces within and around you, and in helping you achieve orgasm is very important. The Prana that moves through breathing makes the body become alive. When breathing is done effectively, the heart opens, the mind becomes calm, and sexual energy starts to flow freely along the spine. When breathing is done incorrectly, it blocks sensations and emotions, as they do not get circulated to the whole body. When breathing is done consciously, it leads to a better connection of mind, body and deepen your partner.

Sex is a sacred meditation, and it shouldn't be done otherwise. Practicing breathing and stillness will help you achieve a higher spiritual consciousness even while making love. Stillness does not mean you would lay still or numb, but it means you will slow down, taking time to relish each moment and each experience.

From the *Eight Limbs of Yoga*, I'm providing a brief explanation of the concept of Pranayama, and how important it is in Yoga and lovemaking. Prana is the short form of the word Pranayama, and it is gotten from two Sanskrit words, *Prana* and *Ayama*. Prana means *life force*, and Ayama means *control*. Basically, it is knowledge of how to control your breath, especially during meditation. Just as the translation of the word itself says, learning to control your breath is vital step towards learning how to control your life force.

Prana is made up of a set of breathing exercises that contain three potential parts:

1. Inhalation (*puraka*)
2. Breath holding (*kumbhaka*)
3. Exhalation (*rechaka*)

We'd all agree that the importance of breathing is something that is always constantly overlooked in our modern society, especially in the West. We are all too in a hurry to pause and take a deep breath. If only we could pay more attention to it, a lot of our physical and psychological problems would be resolved.

The physical nature of things makes it easier for us to see, perceive, examine, and rationalize existence and this can fool us into thinking that everything that matters are visible and concrete.

The truth is, all of life matters and are equally important. The seen and the unseen, the solid and the gaseous, the physical and the spiritual. Our breath is the doorway through which Prana or the force of life enters our body. It travels round the body like an electric power and fuels our life's function by passing through the energy pathways we call *Nadis*. That is why as much as we can stay without food for weeks, water for days, and air for seconds, there's no surviving a microsecond without Prana. There's no life outside of Prana. That's the power of Prana!

The universal measure of life is the breath. Life as we know is made possible by the life force, *the breath of life*. This breath is potent enough to calm the mind, brighten the soul, and heal the heart. The quality of this vital life force can be expanded and improved if we can learn to engage in conscious and free breathing. Pranayama's conscious breathing is about enhancing the quality of this life force.

Pranayama is of great importance to any meditation techniques and Yoga practice, because it's the only function of the body that voluntarily regulated is breathing. If *Prana* means breath of life and *Ayama* means regulation or control, *then Pranayama's acts of voluntary breath control can be the interlink between the mind, body, and spiritual connection.*

Enhanced psychological and physiological functioning is intrinsically connected to refined respiratory movements and optimal breathing. A slow, conscious, suspended, and rhythmic breathing is healing to the mind, body and soul. There's a power with Pranic breathing and we can claim and continue to reclaim it.

Breathing for Kundalini Arousal
(side by side or individual work)

Breathing — to you might not mean much other than an unconscious activity but when you understand it to be the vehicle through which Prana enters and goes around the body, then you will learn to appreciate it and consciously engage in it. The quality of a single breath is very important which is why breathing exercises benefits the body in a lot of ways. It brings about increased energy and the relaxation of the body.

Conscious breathing exercises help to raise Kundalini. This invisible energy is located at the base of the spine. This energy can lie dormant and when it does, it robs us of the ability to carry out its optimal functioning thereby robbing the body of the chance to benefit from its effect.

When awakened, this energy rises from its position at the base of the spine and goes through the whole body by passing through the body's various energy chakras.

Breathing exercises, whether relaxing or energizing, have the potency of awakening the dormant Kundalini. The result of awakened Kundalini, above everything else, is enlightenment and bliss.

The following breathing exercises can awaken the Kundalini. It can be done side by side with your partner or alone by yourself.

In Kundalini Yoga, breathing exercises are from basic to advanced and every practitioner is advised to start from the foundation before attempting to move to the advanced practices. When you master the basic breathing exercises, it will be easier to engage in and master the advance techniques.

The Alternate Nostril Breathing

One of these basic Kundalini breathing exercises is the alternate nostril breathing. The practice of this exercise should involve you taking a seated position and comfortably crossing your legs. Then close your eyes while raising your right hand close to your face. At this position, use your right thumb in pressing your right nostril so it closes.

While still maintaining this position, inhale slowly though your open left nostril. Let it be a long, slow one. Pause and repeat the same thing with your left nostril but this time using the ring finger of your right hand instead of the thumb. Now exhale completely through this open nostril. Spend between 15 and 30 minutes going through this cycle.

Breath of Fire

Compared to the alternate nostril breathing, the breath of fire technique is more invigorating, requiring the use of quick, forceful breaths. This exercise isn't only energizing, it's also cleansing.

Sit comfortably on a chair and begin by doing long and deep inhalation and exhalation. After taking the last inhalation, by contracting the muscles in your abdomen, exhale through your nose, forcing out all the air resident in your lungs.

This movement is always powerful and rapid. Inhale through your nose immediately and let the air fill up your lungs. Repeat this exercise by filling up your lungs and expelling it through the contraction of your abdominal muscles.

Long Deep Breathing

This breathing exercise helps to activate the crown chakra and the third eye, these breaths can be reduced to 4 or less per minutes and 6 or less per minutes respectively.

Lay down comfortably and let the tip of your tongue rest on the roof of your mouth. With your mouth open, inhale through your nose as slowly as possible. Your focus should be on filling up your abdomen for a start, then diaphragm and chest with air. Pause for a short while and repeat the process by exhaling through your nose as slow as you can. Focus on emptying the air in your chest cavity, diaphragm and finally abdomen.

Soham Mantra Breathing

This breathing technique has a way of gradually awakening or activating the Kundalini when it is added to a conscious focus.

Sit comfortably in a cross-legged position. Deeply exhale through the nose and focus on your diaphragm, audibly saying "Hammmm". Deeply inhale while focusing also on the diaphragm, audibly saying "Sooooo". Repeat this breathing technique by doing several cycles of it.

Partner Breathing Practices
(to do together)

This type of breathing practice is done with a partner. There's a healing ability to it when you have another person breathe harmoniously with you. This type of harmonious breathing helps us to develop a sense of oneness, wholeness, or unity in your relationships.

Mirroring Your Partner's Breath

This is powerful breathing technique, and when correctly and effectively done has the power to dissolve tension that you may have held for a long time. It helps you feel more connected to your partner and the bond between you strengthened. It is a profoundly freeing feeling to experience another person mirror your breath.

1. Begin by making eye contact with your partner and acknowledge each other in a silent way.
2. One of you, lay down comfortably on your back and breathe naturally while closing your eyes.
3. Your partner is to observe the movement of your abdomen and match its rhythm to his or her own.
4. After syncing your breathing rhythm, notice how this harmonious breathing makes you feel.
5. Stay in this position as much as it makes you feel connected and comfortable with each other, a few minutes should be enough.
6. After that open your eyes, acknowledge your partner and, without uttering a word, switch places.
7. Let your partner also lie down, close his or her eyes and breathe naturally.
8. You should observe the movement of your partner's abdomen and match his or her rhythm to yours.
9. Notice how the mirroring of your partner's breath makes you feel.
10. Stay in this position for 5 to 10 minutes.

The Aloha Breath

The Aloha breath exercise propagates open-mindedness between partners. After engaging in this exercise, making eye contact with your partner, this becomes more pleasurable; looking into each other's eyes will bring you more together. This practice pushes away aversion, replacing it with a deep sense of connectedness and tranquility. It is a fascinating experience.

1. Begin by standing face-to-face with your partner, acknowledge one another silently using only eye contact, then place your palms together at your hearts.
2. Now lean close to one another so your noses and foreheads are touching.
3. Gaze into one another's eyes and beginning on an exhale, take three deep breaths in harmony.
4. Acknowledge your partner silently, and switch places.

The many stress related problems that abound in our society is because of ignoring our breathing. Prolonged stress and fatigue disrupts our breathing patterns thereby upsetting the balance of the psychological and physiology systems. An important tool to prevent or to remedy this is Pranayama.

It doesn't matter if your goal is to connect with a loved one or you just want to move your energy, breathing exercises have a profound ability to deepen personal relationships. The world will be a better place if occasionally we all learn to practice these breathing exercises. It will heal our wounds, connect us more deeply, and bring us to a state of awesome stillness.

"The body can become a vehicle to that which is beyond body, and sex energy can become a spiritual force."

~ Osho

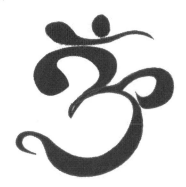

Part 3: Grounding, Stillness, & Integration

CHAPTER 7

"Tantra says, first purify the body – purify it of all repressions. Allow the body energy to flow, remove the blocks. It is very difficult to come across a person who has no blocks, it is very difficult to come across a person whose body is not tight. Loosen this tightness; this tension is blocking your energy, the flow cannot be possible with this tension."

~ Osho

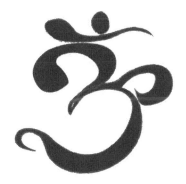

Daily Cultivation

A LOT OF PEOPLE ARE OF THE OPINION THAT TANTRA IS A practice about spiritual sexual union (*and to some extent it is*) but Tantra is much more than sex. The word *"Tantra"* itself actually means the liberation of the body, mind, and spirit. The practice of Tantra helps to liberate all of our realities from societal limitations and constructs so we all can see the sacredness within and behind it all.

It doesn't matter the reason for the blockages and where the blockages are located, a Tantra practice can help you release them, allowing your sexual energy to freely move so you can do all that you are capable of.

Cultivating a Tantric lifestyle, and fully live your life every day. When you inculcate the practice of Tantra into your daily activities, you're conditioning yourself for deeper intimacy, enhanced consciousness, and positivity.

Morning Exercises

With Tantra, we can manifest the reservoir of energy that we have stored inside ourselves. Tantra exercises are geared toward helping to connect us with our emotional bodies, and creating a spiritual balance in the process.

Begin your day on a high by waking up and engage in these Tantric exercises.

1. *Daily Positive Affirmations*

Prepare yourself for the day's activities by making positive affirmations about yourself and what you want your day to look like. Your words shape your world, so why not begin to say what you want your day to be like before you even step into it. It's a great way to prepare yourself for success.

Say these mantras:

"I am enough. I am worthy. I am smart.
I am beautiful inside out.
I am not defeated by the struggles of today.
I come back happy for a fulfilled day.
My work is excellent and I make good decisions today."

Say this while standing in front of your mirror. Say this to yourself when you're faced with a situation that seems bigger than what you can handle. Say it when you think you can't.

2. *Boost Your Energy*

After making positive confirmations, go a step further to energize yourself in preparation for the day's work. This is a natural energy boost:

- Do this by standing up and with your legs 3 feet apart, gently bend over so the tips of your fingers touch the floor.
- If necessary, you can also bend your knees.
- Breathe in as deeply as you can, using your nose, while gradually raising your upper body and head.
- In a controlled manner, breathe out while looking back down and this time with your mouth.

What this exercise will do for you is allow your cerebral spinal fluid to circulate smoothly so you can be fully awake, alert, and refreshed, both mentally and physically.

Evening Exercises

The truth is that practicing Tantra exercises are best carried out any time of day or night. These practices can be successful carried out in a calm moment you choose. Choose a time when you're not in a hurry and in a place where you're less likely to be disturbed.

After the day's work, engage in the following exercise to regain energy for yourself:

1. *Sitale Breath:*

If you desire to obtain inner calm and tranquility, then the Sitale Breath is a wise choice.

- In a comfortable standing or seated position, with your feet placed flat on the floor, breathe in through your mouth and picture your lungs being cleansed by this breath as your rib cage expands.
- Roll your tongue like a funnel while maintaining this position, as a way of cooling the oxygen entering your internal organs.
- Through your nose, let out any discomforts or inhibitions sitting in your chest cavity in the form of stale air.
- Do this for a minimum of three minutes as a way of alleviating stress and setting up yourself for a great night of rest.

2. *Breath of Fire*

The breath of fire exercise is a continuous, diaphragmatic rapid breathing.

- Let your tongue hang out of your mouth, and quickly breathe in and out much like a panting dog.

- This exercise has a way of unbinding uncomfortable feelings, increasing the flow of oxygen, and invigorating the lungs.

Tantra exercises are concerned with deliberate and focused breathing. Deep and intentional inhalation has a way of filling up your lungs with oxygen and in the process revitalizing your energy centers, as it circulates round your body.

Tantra exercise have both physical and metaphysical goals. While your physical goals are invigorated lungs, increased oxygen flow, mental and physical alertness, etc., metaphysical goals are about harmonizing the masculine and feminine sides of our body, awakening or reawakening the Kundalini, and reviving the body's energy centers.

Listening Exercises

Communication is of utmost importance in a relationship. When the communication channels of couples or partners are not open, they can both waste precious time trying to figure out the needs and desires of the other person.

A Tantric communication that is geared towards listening to the other person begins with the creation of a sacred space:

- As partners, sit down across from one another and share an embrace.
- Compliment and bow to one another.
- Set parameters for the exercise. For instance, let one person talk while the other listens for a specific period of time, say 5 or 10 minutes.

- After this time, switch roles. The purpose of this exercise is to learn to not only communicate but also listen in the process.

This communication practice should generally revolve around a question. The question can be about how he or she likes to be touched or kissed. The listener, say partner A, will be the one to ask the question, partner B will then spontaneously respond to the question. Understand that this exercise isn't mainly about conversation but more about knowing something the other person may not have shared before and learning to listen in your relationship.

As the listener, your duty is to listen exclusively, 100 percent. Don't even think about the answers, just listen. When he or she is done with the question, you can then think about how to answer and respond to the question.

At the end of the exercise, embrace and thank each other for their capacity to generously provide the valuable information that was shared.

CHAPTER 8

*"A good orgasm is satisfying, but a great orgasm can be
a revelation of your deepest being, unfolding the truth of
who you are in ecstatic communion with your lover."*

~ David Deida

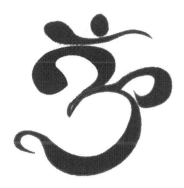

Eroticism

IT SEEMS THE GODS OF LOVE FROM THEIR DIFFERENT traditions and cultures have departed and kissed this world goodbye and are now only consciously viewed as mythical characters in their minds. Or maybe it's the other way around, we sent them packing, removing every semblance of their presence and nature, *which is love,* not only from the temples but also from our hearts.

By sending them packing, we have also succeeded in causing the disappearance of their energy from the face of the Earth, leading to serious confusion as the role of eroticism in human existence.

The result of this confusion lead to the distortion of eroticism to the point of it being giving a strictly sexual meaning has led to the situation where the relationship between a man and a woman, or human to human, is now based on sexuality and of the satisfaction of sexual urges. It is now only linked to sex, sexuality or even pornography.

What people fail to understand is that eroticism and Eros goes beyond sex to the place of bodily unification. Couples are intended to "make love" and not "have sex" because while sex gradually diminishes the love existing in a relationship to the point where it is only sexual and instinctual, lovemaking strengthens relationships because it attracts the Divine energy of Eros.

Sex and sexuality separates, isolates us in the limitation of our ego and confines us to our animal nature, a place where our only concern is survival. At this level of inferior human nature, we are saturated with a compulsive thirst for pleasure, particularly a personal one. Couples ruled by sex or sexuality will seek dominate or possess each other, and their desire will be the achievement of pleasure. The relationship will most likely suffer, decay, discord, and an eventual destruction to the point of breakup.

Eroticism and Eros on the other hand has a primordial energy which is directed in opposite direction to what sex or sexuality does. This energy which is intimately linked to the energy of love is one of unification. No matter the individuals level of sexual experience, there can always be an erotic energy between them. When awakened, this energy seeks to strengthen and purify the bond of relationships and its impregnation with a state of sacredness. The very essence of eroticism and Tantra is the spiritual transformation of sex.

The key to a longer and more powerful orgasmic experience during lovemaking is the building of this energy. And we routinely practice this erotic energy, it aligns with other areas of our lives like intimacy, relationship, and spirituality.

The attitude and disposition of Tantra towards eroticism and sexuality is very practical, uninhibited, spiritual, and loving. It encourages and inspires you to wholly embrace life and say yes to it. Tantra teaches that all of life are connected and becomes united ultimately.

People make the mistake of thinking that sexuality and eroticism are the same thing, that cannot be farther from the truth. The reason why people would think they are the same is simple, the world revolves around sex, and the idea of achieving orgasm and fast as possible. People no longer pay attention to the body of their partner or the idea of sensuality. In Tantra, these things are important, and eroticism is the core. I have explained that sex is never just sex, it is more fully described as making love, and it is the practice of releasing energy and merging them.

It is important to first understand the difference between sexuality and eroticism before you can know the processes of achieving eroticism. The purpose of eroticism transcends sex, it is meant to connect you and your partner on a deeper level. If it were to be only sex, then there would be no difference between humans and animals; sex is a natural urge. Tantra helps you take it beyond just the natural urge to the level where it becomes spiritual. It is not about the number of minutes or the number of positions you use, it is about what you and your partner bring to the experience; the emotion, the passion, the *dharana* focus, and the *dhyana* or meditative absorption.

Female Eroticism

The human body is dynamic. Each gender has a different sex centers, these centers are what drives our pleasure and it is the point of concentration in the body.

In the body of the woman, erotic activities are best activated by starting and focusing on the circumference of her body. You can put your hands on her shoulder and knee, this creates a feeling of safety and trust for her. This can be followed by holding her belly in a state of pure presence, doing this will help her open-up the sacral chakra and emotional fluidity.

The female nipples have nerves that link to the clitoris, when the breasts are sensitively massaged, your partner can be able to access a deeper kind of sexual arousal. Honoring the third eye is also an amazing way of achieving a good erotic love play with your partner. The third eye is part of the energy map of the chakras, massage it through the forehead, starting between the eyebrows to the hairline. This will awaken her Goddess nature, and allow a fluid flow of emotions and love. Honoring her third eye will make her feel safe and fluid.

In the body of a woman, starting slowly and then moving gradually towards the sex center is very important. Your approach shouldn't be direct, instead, it should be teasing and inviting. If the man approaches the woman's yoni with honor and reverence, the woman would fully surrender to him and her ecstasy would know no bound.

The issue of female eroticism is as misunderstood as Tantra itself. The issue of female eroticism is encompassed by so much misinformation that it becomes confusing trying to understand it. Is there a socially acceptable way that women are expected to portray their eroticism. How are they expected to be their natural sexual self? How should they embody their sexuality? How should the incredible potential of their female sexuality be represented? These and other are the questions begging for answers as it relates to female eroticism.

A woman's sexual power isn't only domiciled in her genitals. A woman's sexuality is holistic, affecting her senses, emotions, and her erogenous zones. Therefore, it said that a woman possesses emotional fluidity. When it comes to orgasmic ecstasy and sexual fulfilment for women, the place of emotional fluidity is of significant importance. This fluidity makes it possible for women to access a deeper level of intimacy and heightened sensitivity. Emotional flow and sexual pleasure, for women, are interrelated directly.

Unluckily for the women, no one came with a manual on how to make use of her sexuality. No pre-knowledge of what making love, having pleasure, or having a fulfilling relationship involves. We were just thrown into this world and expected to just know all these things. So since we do not come fitted with the knowledge of how to handle our eroticism, our best bet is to learn how, and this is where Tantra comes in.

Tantra says to us, instead of expecting other people to know what you need exactly to bring you sexual fulfilment, compartmentalizing your sexuality, accepting what others think is feminism or sexuality and how it should be expressed, it is far better for you to find out the answer yourself, from deep within. We cannot expect people who do not know us to understand us and tell us exactly what we need. We have to understand that a joyous and fulfilled life is largely dependent on a healthy sexuality. A healthy sexuality is concerned with the integration of emotions with the spirit.

Hidden in a woman's body is an immense orgasmic potential. Every part of her body, from her voice, breasts; to her touch, is an ocean of intimacy and unrivalled pleasure. She is an instrument of joy and pleasure.

As against its reputation of being only sexual, Tantric sex, sacred sexuality, is much more than eye contact, breathing, and marathon orgasms. Tantric sex is about delaying gratification, it's about delaying sexual releases, and prioritizing emotional release and sensory pleasure.

As perceived by Tantra, sex is a spiritual act, and it leads to more awareness of one's body, whether it's in the bedroom or outside of it. Tantric sex is way beyond sex and when engaged in with an open heart and mind, the result will not only be improved and better sex but also deeper connection between partners, and better intimate communication.

Tantric sex is about self-awareness, mindfulness, and the willingness to listen to your body and how it responds to sensation and touch. It's about your connection to your body, soul, and spirit. It's about a deeper connection!

Male Eroticism

Eroticism with men is slightly different from what it is with women. With the man, it is better to start right with the lingam, honoring the lingam of the man first sets him in the right mood. The first thing is to get him aroused, and for him to feel his potency. After this, you can the spread the sexual energy that you have stirred up all over his body. To spread the sexual energy, you can start by stroking down his legs down to his feet, then to his shoulders, his hands, and so on. Only when the lingam has been honored should you attempt to go to other areas of the body.

It is important to understand how eroticism works in both the male and female body. It is in understanding this disparity that partners can really get the best out of their experiences. Unfortunately, people are not paying attention to this, a lot of men treat their women as they – *the men*, would like to be treated, not considering the distinct need of women. This happens with women too, as a lot of women treat men the way they – *the women*, would like to be treated. With this approach, people just focus on the intercourse and not the process of exploring each other's body.

Right from the start of their sexual voyage, men have been conditioned to view sex in a certain way. This conditioning makes it seems like thy are not meant to experience deeper pleasure. This type of conditioning is responsible for the ejaculation mindset. The ejaculation mindset is all about "getting it on" and "getting it over with" right from adolescent till old age. From the stage of being boys to when they became men, men were never schooled on what the sacredness of their sexuality really mean. They never got the chance to understand what being a healthy sexuality male entails.

This conditioning and a lack of the knowledge of what is truly possible makes accepting that there's much more to their sexual experience a difficult thing. They had already been addicted to the ejaculation mindset, and to them the ultimate sexual experience was ejaculation, nothing more.

The pornography industry hasn't helped matter with their insistence on the area of masculine performance and capping it up by "coming," further distorting male eroticism. What the man must understand is that there's so much more than the norm of ejaculation. You just must choose to see what's beyond what you now believe to be the height of sexual pleasure. Instead of the normal ejaculatory orgasm, you can experience full body orgasm. You can get to the point of no return where you will enjoy your pleasurable orgasm over and over again in a single moment.

How do you move beyond the normal and get to the point of no return? Begin by engaging in breathing techniques at the point of ejaculation. When you get close to the point of no return during lovemaking, pause for a little while, take three to four deep breaths and focus on what you are feeling in your body, in your genitals.

When you do this, you will notice the intensity of your pleasure relaxing and moving away from your genitals, thereby spreading this pleasure up the spine and around the body. Start again and keep repeating it. The more you engage in this practice the more this sexual pleasure spreads until it takes over your entire being.

Start by being aware of what is going on inside your body and as this awareness of how the sexual energy spreads through your body increases, the more aware you will be of the difference between orgasm and ejaculation. Your ability to make this distinction will uplift your sex life in more ways than one. As you focus on this difference and choosing to bring the intensity of the ejaculation forward, stopping and then breathing, you will be further expanding that intensity into unknown orgasmic pleasure.

Your Loving Sanctuary

Women have been conditioned to view sex as something to be ashamed of. To desire for more pleasure is sometimes viewed as a sign of promiscuity and lewdness. The men have been so schooled in the art of ejaculatory orgasm that it's very difficult convincing them that there's something else than orgasms induced by ejaculation.

The awareness of the true capabilities of both man and woman opens something huge and magical in them. A feeling of limitlessness, the feeling that there's no more boundaries, the feeling of unlimited ecstasy. You see yourself in your own loving sanctuary.

> Tantric sex is empowering and energizing. It's the sanctuary within. It's like lying on the sand of the world's best beach and savoring its beauty while soaking in the bliss of the beautiful ocean wave. The sensation is electrifying and the pleasure endless. It's like shooting into timelessness... everything else freezes and ceases to exist except you in the arms of your pleasure. It's the store of cosmic orgasm and pure euphoria...the state of heightened ecstasy. Tantric sex is LOVE.

Tantra tells us to breath in the pleasure of our sexual energy, to let go of all expectations and enjoy the present moment. Tantra teaches us to untangle our love life, sexual power, and romance and by so doing, to reveal the hidden mysteries of our innermost nature. We are to embrace the limitations of our lives and so step on the path of awareness of the secrets that lies within us. Dehumanizing routines is replaced with ecstatic experiences, and uninspiring and mechanical sex metamorphosed into intimate bliss for our lives and those of our loved ones.

Whether you agree or not, the topic of eroticism affects our everyday life. Nearly all adverts are geared towards manipulating the people's subconscious continuously and stimulating their instinctual desires. The promise of a later fulfilment produces an unquenchable thirst in people.

But the journey towards sexual pleasure doesn't have to end in clitoral or ejaculatory orgasms, there's so much that can be done. When rightly exercised, male and female eroticism, apart from improved sexual life, can also lead to the healing of deep-seated wounds, the release of shame, and bring about deeper connection between partners.

CHAPTER 9

Feelings come and go like clouds in a windy sky.
Conscious breathing is my anchor.

~ Thích Nhất Hạnh

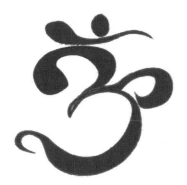

Coming Home
Together

OUR NATURE AS HUMANS HAS LIMITED US SEXUALLY
in certain ways, one of which is the difference in the way and manner
with which orgasm and pleasure is experienced in males and females.
Pleasure and orgasm for men during sex is always in the timeframe of
minutes and going an hour for the average man is almost impossible

because it would require them to exercise strong mental and muscle control so as to prevent their basic nature of going through ejaculatory orgasms in minutes, but this is quite different for women.

Women are naturally more suited to enjoy pleasure and orgasms when sexual activity lasts longer. Men are easily aroused and it doesn't take long for them to reach their climax while women take them longer time to get aroused and reach climax. And there's nothing better than when sex is both enjoyed by the participating couple instead of by only one of the two parties involved.

This difference in sexual orientation if not understood and properly managed may lead to broken relationships and marriages. As a result, men must come to the realization that sex isn't a one-way ticket but rather a two-way co-creation. They also have to understand that getting it on and releasing it isn't the only way to have orgasms. There's more pleasure when you hold back your orgasm and seek to please your partner so that she can also reach her own orgasm.

The truth is that men are not educated on this, just like I said in the beginning, but with a strong willpower, it is achievable. This position isn't only for the men; the women too have a role to play. They too can learn to regulate their arousal in a way that it closely matches that of their partner.

Tantra provides us with the tools to help them find an equilibrium point where they can reduce their sexual speed and connect with the arousal level of one another. This will move them towards becoming more sexually intuitive. Tantric sex isn't about having prolonged sex, it's the practice of sexual mindfulness.

The practice of Tantric sex is to prolong penetration and thereby prolong orgasm so as to build true mental and physical excitement. The use of meditations, breathing techniques, genital and non-touching foreplay are the tools employed in Tantric practice to cause sex an in-the-moment, fun, and highly satisfying experience rather than one where the only pleasure comes at the point of ejaculation.

The Union of Love & Meditation

Tantra is a spiritual path unlike its ascribed sexual exploration tag, although there's nothing wrong with sexual exploration, which also makes it a sexual path.

One fundamental principle in Tantra is that of transcendence. It is believed that the union of opposites can lead to the attainment of transcendence. These opposites are known as Yin and Yang in Taoism and are represented in nature as fire and water, night and day, heaven and Earth, male and female. In Tantra, these opposites are known as Shiva and Shakti.

According to *Osho*, Tantra is the union of love and meditation, and while love is the Shakti part, meditation is the Shiva part. In everyday life, Shakti predominates and the individual can easily get lost in his or her experiences majorly because it is the part we sense, feel, and experience, as against Shiva which is the part that witnesses and sees that which is experienced. Shakti's predomination is because of too much identification with each thought or experience.

> While the monastic life chooses meditation over love because it elevates meditative awareness while reducing external experience, Tantra chooses the union of both meditation and love. Tantra as a spiritual path is practiced because a lot of the spiritual paths is related to the monastic way.

The problem with Tantra is practitioners laying more emphasis on the experiences while relegating meditation to the background. Common among new entrants of Tantra practice is the rush for experience while neglecting the meditative practice.

Over-identification of experiences produces emotional dysfunction, confusion, and chaos. The Tantric attachment to experience may cause the individual to long for the repeat of the experience. The result of this is an overwhelming pain of desire. The effects can be balanced with a simple meditation. Over identification with meditation also has its own downside because meditation without a balanced mixture of experience may become withdrawn, stiff, and lacking in empathy.

Tantra is about balancing both. While the feminine practice dances opens the individual to life, the masculine practice of meditation and Tantric study connects one to consciousness.

Breathing Tantra Meditations

Tantric meditation is different from the other forms of meditation in that it seeks to awaken consciousness as a mean of liberating Shakti energy, as opposite most yogic meditation which seeks to achieve relaxation and tranquility, as commonly practiced in the West.

The misinterpretation of Tantra meditation and practices has been particularly made worse by the West with their associating it with spiritual sexuality, saying that sex has a way of elevating the practitioner to a higher spiritual plane. But from its Sanskrit meaning where "*tan*" means expansion and "*tra*" means liberation, Tantra meditation is concerned with expanding the mind and activating consciousness.

There's an energy of Tantra where the only thing you feel is the saturating flow of Divine's energy as it floods your body, freeing you from all resentment. This feeling is possible and it can be a regular, non-stop feeling once there's an unlocking or unblocking of kundalini.

What is this Kundalini?

Kundalini is a coil of pure energy, *visualized as a snake and known as a serpent*, residing at the base of the spine. This tightly coiled energy can be unlocked and moved up through the spine, passing through the other energy centers, and finally uniting with the crown chakra.

Kundalini can be unlocked through Tantra meditation and the chakras are also activated so that the freed Shakti can move from the root chakra all the way to the crown chakra. By setting this energy free, consciousness is awakened and the whole body is also awakened. This energy can also be directed from the head or crown chakra back to the root chakra.

The techniques of Tantra meditations are designed in such a way that visualization, breath work, mantras, sacred geometry, and music are employed not only to speed up and encourage the process of linking the kundalini from the root to the crown but also to amplify its energy and effectiveness. Group Tantra meditation is believed to increase the effectiveness of the kundalini.

Kundalini energy can be contained and harvested with the appropriate Tantra meditation techniques. When done, it brings about wholesome connection in the body and a higher level of power in all areas of your everyday life.

Don't make the mistake of thinking that you can find a sexual release for this energy because if you do, it will only leave you tired and exhausted, and instead of being invigorated, you'll be dispirited. So, if you truly want to maximize and bring to surface this dormant energy lying inside of you, then Tantra meditation is your best option. You can change your life and improve your world in more areas than one.

Raising Spiritual Consciousness

To most people, Tantra is a means to pleasure and fun, and even though I do not see anything wrong in that, that opinion is a one-sided approach because it overlooks the cosmic essence and energetic power of sex that is available to us as conscious beings. A lot can be gained, as it doesn't matter if it has to do with pleasure or not, what matters more is depth. The deeper you go, the higher you go.

In their study of the path to enlightenment, Tantra masters discovered that of the many different forms of energy, the sexual energy is very potent and that is why Tantra focuses on it — not for any other ascribed reasons. The Tantra practitioners of old discovered that through the use of sexual energy found in the natural world, they could reach or access the spiritual world beyond.

A look into the inherent character of orgasm showed that it can a tool for meditation. A deeper study of this force of nature revealed incredible details: it is possible to meditate during orgasm, and orgasm on its own is a form of enlightenment. The average individual misses out on the opportunity to discover this transcendence aspect of orgasm because it happens too fast, i.e. the time is too short.

Orgasm for a lot of us, both male and female, is a fleeting experience. It happens so fast that the only thing they can remember of it is, its amazing part. Since Tantra teachers have discovered the inherent power of the sexual energy resident in orgasm, they decided to find ways to contain and harvest this power. One of such ways is to prolong this period of transcendence from the normal seconds to several minutes. It can even be for an hour or hours. We can reach into the Divine via our orgasm in as much as an hour.

What Tantra did, was make it possible for us to see into the Divine for a longer time than normal so the person can bask in the euphoria of this enlightened state, and all we need to do is take some simple steps. These steps involve a reduction in the speed at which the sexual activity is going, becoming more aware of, and feeling the sexual energy, increasing the duration of the sexual activity, being in control of the sexual energy, and being able to direct it.

The wave of orgasm can be ridden through Tantric practices. This wave of orgasm, unlike the quick peaking orgasm from the genitals that most people are used to, begins like a surge of blissful pleasure, and a feeling of oneness and unity with your partner and the Divine. It doesn't stop there, it goes deeper and as it does, the pleasure is heightened and you're floating on the spiritual wave of ecstatic pleasure.

Multiple groundbreaking and soul-shaking orgasms can be achieved through Tantra and the partners will come out feeling very different, like the divinity has rubbed off on them, like they've been touched by the Divine. The experience is a shift in consciousness becomes yours, the feeling that you can almost touch God.

Nearly all of us grew up with the conditioned belief that there's no correlation between spirituality and sex, but unknown to us are a lot of practices to support the interrelatedness of both of them. For thousands of years, sex has been employed as means of attaining more connection, more mindfulness, and increased consciousness.

An elevated state of consciousness is experienced during Tantric sex. Sexual activity also draws and bonds the participating couples together. Meditation and other practices like breathing, non-touching arousal, etc. can enhance your physical sensations and emotions, and improve your awareness during Tantric sex.

This Tantric sex is firmly founded on a Tantric philosophy which states that the sexual energy in our body can be employed as a means of accessing a higher spiritual state.

About the Author

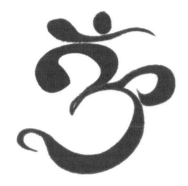

Rishi Eric Infanti

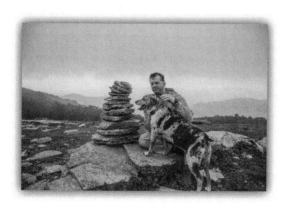

Praised Yoga teacher & transformational coach, Rishi Eric Infanti presents another work in his inter-web of publications, *Adornment – Awakening the Conscious Man: Walking the Tantric Path*. This body of work radiates your relationship to self and others through the understanding and practice of Tantra & Yoga and where they intersect beneath the veil of illusion — in a brilliant and extraordinary new light.

Rishi embarks upon an extraordinary new volume. *Adornment – Awakening the Conscious Man* provides a deeply practical prescription for heightening your sexuality, healing past trauma and deepening your sense of connection.

Infanti's previous books and online courses of guided wisdom — *Marine on the Mat*, *Breath Becomes Life*, *Yoga for the Martial Way*, and *Mindfulness & Yin Yoga*, earns a global following for their uniqueness, depth and intimate spiritual insight.

Now, Infanti continues his teachings with this widely awaited new imprint. *Adornment – Awakening the Conscious Man* leads you through a wholly new consideration of your relationship with yourself and partnership, bringing you to your highest expression through the understanding Tantra, specifically Tantra where it intersects the connection to self, relationship as well as the Divine.

Adornment – Awakening the Conscious Man harmoniously helps the reader develop as spiritual beings within while living an increasingly sexual, high-spirited, and self-assured Tantric practitioners, amid the pressures of outward life. Filled with Tantric exercises, Yoga, and affirming to both practitioners and teachers alike, *Adornment – Awakening the Conscious Man* immediately produces transformation in the life of every aspiring conscious lover who approaches it.

Perfect for Tantric teachers and new practitioners alike, this book is an extraordinary experience in a new body of guided wisdom that is attracting readers across the globe.

A U.S. Marine Corps veteran, Rishi is a teacher of Iyengar, Ashtanga, Vinyasa and Yin Yoga. She has studied in Mysore, India with Sri K. Pattabhi Jois's family at the Ashtanga Yoga Research Institute and Acharya V. Sheshadri. His background and training include over 2,000 hours of Yoga Teacher Training and has been exploring the psychology of the mind - body connection to foster balance and equanimity, while deepening his passion for movement and contemplation to form his own constitution.

Rishi is a gifted therapist, Transformational Mindset & Marketing Coach for Therapists, Alternative Healers & Yoga Teachers, he is the creator of the Mela Academy Mastery Coaching Program, helping Alternative professionals & studios rapidly grow their businesses through mindset and marketing execution.

Rishi takes his experience and vast amount of knowledge to another level, thus implementing online education and business marketing services to the ever-growing health, wellness and fitness industry. Trained as a Software Project Manager and Systems' Analyst, Rishi has now designed marketing and technology-related programs, products and services aimed to educate the next generation of healers and trainers by providing them with strategic tooling necessary to compete in today's dynamic marketplace.

It is from this template that he leads a Yoga practice into a calm and focused style of instruction, allowing each student to fully access the practice. Yet, it is from a space of love and compassion that he works with others to bring Yoga into all areas of life as a vehicle for wellness, healing and personal transformation.

It is Rishi's passion to help people and their canine counterparts to recover their health and live at an optimal state. As a multi-modality professional, he has the unique ability to quickly identify and treat issues at a variety of levels of being. She has extensive experience with severe physical injuries and ailments while working with high performance athletes to aging seniors.

A Jiu-Jitsu Brown Belt, and therapist of a myriad of over 30 modalities, he is board certified in Therapeutic Massage & Bodywork working primarily in Sport, Neuromuscular and Deep Tissue, is trained in Ayurveda, energy work and Thai Massage, while straddling both body therapy and traditional physical therapy to heal complex biomechanical issues.

Rishi is a certified personal trainer, a tactical fitness instructor and a CrossFit Level 2 Coach, holding seven additional CrossFit certifications. She has been the therapist for, coached and trained a more diverse group of people than ever imagined, from a team of world-class athletes, to aspiring competitors, to seniors of a maturing audience with highly complex physiological and clinical issues.

His approach is an eclectic methodology to facilitate healthy awareness, rooted in creativity, movement, and meditation as the medium of personal change and transformation. She facilitates this by holding con-text for optimal wellness, participant safety, and mindfulness; tailored to fit personal and group needs to utilize the replenishing mind-body-spirit modalities through creative expression. These practices are skillfully blended to serve participants in optimizing their wellness, empowering all life stages, and assimilating their life experiences within a fitness setting.

Rishi is a graduate of The New England Institute for Transforming Consciousness with a Master's Degree of Consciousness studies in Ayurveda; with a concentration in the Advanced Ayurveda Bodywork and Spirituality, and Union Institute and University with a Master's Degree in Buddhist and Transpersonal Psychology, focusing in spiritually oriented contemplative healing modalities from Hindu and Buddhist philosophies as they intersect with Western psychology.

Rishi is available for workshops, trainings and seminars on Tantra, the Business of Yoga, eclectic Yoga Asana programs, Yoga Teacher Trainings, Yoga Philosophy, and integrating the Eight Limbs of Yoga into your Yoga classes; as well as CrossFit Mobility, Kettlebell, Olympic Lifting, and how to integrate CrossFit into both every day and military lifestyles. To book Rishi, contact him at: eric@MelaAcademy.com.

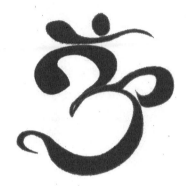

Tantra Journal

Tantra & Yoga Journal:

1. Determine your current Yoga, breathing & fitness status & level. Take some time to assess where you are, take inventory to help you see where you want to go next with your Yoga & Pranayama practice.

Below, briefly describe your current Yoga, breathing & fitness status and activity level. What types of Yoga, breath-work, and physical activity do you currently engage in? At what intensity and for how long? If you've been to Yoga classes or private sessions, or have performed formal fitness testing as part of a wellness or health course, include a summary of the results below.

Description of current Yoga & fitness activity & exercise habits:

Results you are getting from these activities:

Are you satisfied with your current activity and levels? Why or why not?

Tantra Journal Notes:

Made in the USA
Columbia, SC
27 July 2024

39403511R00117